Baby
Names

From Aisha to
Zander, Mary
to Robert ... All
the Names You'll
Ever Need

Carol McD. Wallace

Collins
An Imprint of HarperCollinsPublishers

HarperCollins books may be purchased for educa-
tional, business, or sales promotional use. For information please write: Special Markets Department,
HarperCollins Publishers, 10 East 53rd Street, New York,
NY 10022.

FIRST EDITION

Designed by Emily Cavett Taff

ISBN-10: 0-06-089105-X

ISBN-13: 978-0-06-089105-3

06 07 08 09 10 ❖ / WOR 10 9 8 7 6 5 4 3 2 1

abbreviations

Af	African	*Ir. Gael*	Irish Gaelic
Arab	Arabic	*It*	Italian
Celt	Celtic	*Jap*	Japanese
Dan	Danish	*Lat*	Latin
Eng	English	*Lith*	Lithuanian
Fem	Feminization of	*ME*	Middle English
Fr	French	*Nig*	Nigerian
Gael	Gaelic	*Nor*	Norwegian
Gk	Greek	*OE*	Old English
Haw	Hawaiian	*OF*	Old French
Heb	Hebrew	*OG*	Old German
Hung	Hungarian	*ONorse*	Old Norse

Per	Persian
Pol	Polish
Port	Portuguese
Rus	Russian
Scan	Scandinavian
Scot	Scottish
Scot. Gael.	Scottish Gaelic
Sp	Spanish
Teut	Teutonic

introduction

How many options do you need to find exactly the right name for your baby? This book is a condensation of a much longer volume, *20,001 Names for Baby*. When my sister was pregnant for the first time, we went through that entire book to make a short list of potential choices. After considering the thousands of names I'd collected, we could only find three candidates, none of which she used.

Which made me wonder, why use a baby name book at all? Why not just sift through all the names you can think of and make a list of possibilities?

The answer came to me pretty fast: because you can't think of all the names. You're bound to forget some of the good ones. And chances are, you'll need more possibilities than you thought. The second time I got pregnant, my husband and I knew we were having a son. We liked the idea of a

family name and remembered a great-uncle named
Hugh. So after the baby was born, the orderly was
taking me down to my room at 3:00 A.M. and said,
"What's the baby's name?"

"Hugh," I answered proudly.

"What?" he said.

"Hugh. His name's Hugh," I answered, a little
testy.

"You? You named your baby 'you?'"

Needless to say, our son had a new name by
dawn, but I sure wished I'd packed a baby name
book in my hospital bag.

I tell this story to make clear that naming a baby
is not a scientific process. You do need lots of possible choices and you do need a book to remind
you of potential options you've forgotten. The
virtue of this book is its compactness. I know as
that ninth month ticks by any extra weight you're
carrying will feel like an imposition, so I see this
as a big plus. And though lots of other baby name
books offer many times more possibilities, you've
got plenty here. To bring *20,001 Names* down to
this size, I took out some of the more unusual
choices and trimmed down the number of variants I offered. Often these were just new phonetic

spellings. For this book I limited myself to a few of those and a few international variants, but there are still well over 5,000 names here.

Of course, having been in the baby name business since 1990, I have opinions and observations on the subject and this is my chance to share them.

1. Boys are harder to name than girls. For some reason, we're still more conservative about boys' names. I don't want to think too much about why this is, but it seems okay to give a girl a traditionally male name, whereas you very rarely see a name going the other way. Parents may make up a name for a girl or adopt a word that has not traditionally been a name (Sierra, anyone?), but they wouldn't do that for a boy. The names here are divided almost evenly between girls' and boys' options, but the boys' selections are more traditional.

2. Beware of the trendy name. Some names are standards and stay well used for years on end. Others go into and out of fashion in a kind of long curve, whereas others are simply rare. But the names that will sound

dated are the ones that shoot into popularity out of nowhere. The U.S. government maintains a wonderful website (http://www.ssa.gov/OACT/babynames/index.html) that allows you to check the popularity of any given name. You really don't want to saddle your child with a name that is going to be passé ten years from now.

3. Think hard about the most popular names. Carol was hugely fashionable the year I was born. In most gatherings of more than twenty women, there will be at least two of us in the room. I don't like this.

4. Consider the unusual name pretty carefully, too. Your child may not enjoy the constant confusions or explanations. "Actually, I'm named after the city where I was conceived" has always struck me as more than I want to know about someone.

5. The middle name gives you a place to put something a little less user-friendly, like a slightly peculiar family name. Just watch the initials so that they don't spell out an awkward three-letter word.

You should be able to find a wonderful name for your baby here, even though this book is small. But if you want more options or more information, maybe you should turn to the original version, *20,001 Names for Baby,* or even the expanded edition, *The Greatest Baby Name Book Ever.* In the end, you're sure to find exactly the right name for the newest member of your family.

A

Abelia (*Fem.* **Abel**) *Fr.* from *Heb.* "Sigh."
> **Abella, Abelle**

Abia *Arab.* "Great."

Abida *Arab.* "She who worships"; *Heb.* "My father knows."

Abigail *Heb.* "My father is joyful." Biblical name adopted by the Puritans and popular throughout the 18th century. Later revived with the trend toward old-fashioned names beginning in the 1970s.
> **Abagail, Abbe, Abbey, Abby, Abigal, Abigayle, Avichayil, Gael, Gayle**

Abijah *Heb.* "God is my father."
> **Abisha**

Abra (*Fem.* **Abraham**) *Heb.* "Father of many"; *Arab.* "Example, lesson." King Solomon's favorite concubine was named Abra.

Acacia *Gk.* Name of a blossoming tree that symbolized resurrection. Derivatives such as **Casey** occur often in the United States.

> Casey, Cassie, Kassy

Ada *Ger.* "Noble, nobility." Originated as a short form of names such as **Adelaide** and popular in the last quarter of the 19th century, though infrequently used now.

> Adda, Adia

Adalia *Heb.* "God is my refuge"; *OG.* "Noble one." *See also* **Adelaide**.

> Adal, Adala

Adara *Gk.* "Beauty"; *Arab.* "Virgin."

> Adra

Addie Diminutive of **Adelaide**, **Adeline**, or **Addison**. A nostalgic-sounding nickname.

> Addy

Addison *OE.* "Son of Adam." Climbing the ranks of popularity as a girl's name, probably influenced by the trendy Madison.

> Addeson, Adisson

Adelaide *OG.* "Noble, nobility." First popular in England after the reign (1830–1837) of William IV and Queen Adelaide. The city of Adelaide, Australia, founded in 1836, was named for her.

> Adalayde, Addie, Adela, Adelaida, Adeline,
> Adelle, Aline, Della, Edeline, Eline, Heidi

Adena *Heb.* "Decoration."
> Adina, Deena

Adeola *Nig.* "Crown."

Adiba *Arab.* "Cultured, refined."
> Adeeba, Adibah

Adira *Heb.* "Noble, powerful."
> Adeera, Edira

Aditi *Hindi.* "Boundless." In Hindu cosmology, Aditi is the
mother of the gods.

Adoncia *Sp.* "Sweet."
> Doncia

Adora *Lat.* "Adored."
> Adorabelle, Adorée

Adrian *Lat.* Place name: Adria was a North Italian city. First
popular in the 1950s in Britain, and more common as a
boy's name.
> Adria, Adriana, Adrienne

Agate *OF.* A semiprecious stone. The agate, though not a
particularly beautiful stone, was once believed to have
numerous magical and curative powers.

Agatha *Gk.* "Good." Saint Agatha was a 3rd-century Christian
who refused to marry a Roman consul. She was tortured
and ultimately martyred. Her name was popular in the early
years of the Christian Church and again in the late 19th
century.
> Agata, Agathe, Agota

Agnes *Gk.* "Pure, virginal." Another early Christian saint's name. She was a virgin martyr, and her emblem in art is a lamb (the Latin for "lamb" is *agnus*). Very popular in England between the 12th and 16th centuries.

> Agnella, Agnese, Agneta, Anaïs, Annice, Ines, Nessa, Oona, Senga, Una, Ynez

Ahava *Heb.* "Loved one."

> Ahouva, Ahuva, Ahuda

Aida *Arab.* "Reward, present." Name of an immensely popular opera by Giuseppe Verdi.

> Aeeda, Ayeeda, Aleeda,

Aidan *Ir. Gael.* "Fire." Saint Aidan was a 7th-century Irish monk. The name is used substantially more often for boys than for girls.

> Aiden, Aydan

Aiko *Jap.* "Little loved one."

Aileen *Ir. Gael.* Variation of **Helen** (*Gk.* "Light"). This form has been most popular in Scotland.

> Ailene, Alene, Aline

Ailsa *Scot.* The name has two possible sources. As a homonym for **Elsa**, a diminutive of **Elizabeth**, it means "pledge from God." An alternate source is the tiny Scottish island Ailsa Craig.

> Ailis, Elsa

Aimée *Fr.* "Beloved." *See also* **Amy.**

> Aimie, Aimey, Amey, Amie

Ainsley *Scot. Gael.* Place name: "one's own meadow." A last name converted to a first name, used by both sexes.
>**Ainslee, Ainsleigh, Ainslie, Aynsley**

Aisha *Arab.* "Woman"; *Swahili.* "Life." Aisha was the favored wife of Mohammed; hence the name's current popularity among Muslim families.
>**Aeesha, Aesha, Aeshah, Aiesha, Ashah, Ayeesha, Ayisha, Ieasha, Ieeshia, Yiesha**

Aiyana *Native American.* "Forever flowering."

Akela *Haw.* "Noble." A form of **Adele.**

Alaia *Arab.* "Sublime."

Alanna (*Fem.* **Alan**) *Ir. Gael.* "Rock" or "comely." Also a possible derivative of **Elaine** (*OF.* "Bright, shining") or **Helen** (*Gk.* "Light").
>**Alaina, Alaine, Alanis, Alannah, Alayne, Alène, Allena, Allyn, Lana, Lannah**

Alaula *Haw.* "Light of daybreak."

Alberta *OE.* "Noble shining." Rare and old-fashioned now, it was most widely used during the lifetime of Queen Victoria's prince consort, Albert. Also the name of a western Canadian province and a very popular strain of peach.
>**Alberthine, Albertina, Alli, Berry, Berta, Elberta, Elberthina**

Albinia (*Fem.* **Alban, Albin**) *Lat.* "White, fair."
>**Alba, Albina, Alva**

Alcina *Gk.* In Greek mythology, a sorceress who ruled over a magical island. When she tired of her lovers, Alcina turned them into animals, trees, or stones. Despite this startling role model, the name occurs from time to time.

Alcinia, Alsina

Aldara *Gk.* "Winged gift."

Aldonza *Sp.* "Sweet."

Aleeza *Heb.* "Joy."

Aleczah, Alieza, Alizah

Alegria *Sp.* "Happiness, joy." For related names, *see* **Bliss; Felicia; Hillary; Joy.** A charming choice for a much-wanted child.

Allegria

Aleta *Gk.* "Footloose."

Aletta

Alexandra (*Fem.* **Alexander**) *Gk.* "Man's defender." Became very popular in Britain after the prince of Wales (later Edward VII) married the Danish princess Alexandra in 1863. Still current in the English royal family and its many branches. Both this form and Alexander are very well used in the United States.

Alejandra, Alejandrina, Aleka, Alessandra, Alessandrine, Alessia, Alex, Alexa, Alexandrina, Alexis, Alix, Alla, Allessa, Ally, Lexie, Sanda, Sandie, Sandrine, Sasha, Sohndra, Xandra

Alexis *Gk.* "Helper." Usually thought of as a short form of
  Alexandra, though it has a different etymological root.
>   Alessi, Alexa, Alexia, Lexy

Alfreda (*Fem.* **Alfred**) *OE.* "Elf/power."
>   Alfre, Alfreeda, Alfrieda, Elfrida, Elva, Fredy,
>   Frieda

Alice *OG.* "Noble, nobility." An old standby name since the
  Middle Ages that became enormously popular after the
  1865 publication of Lewis Carroll's *Alice's Adventures in
  Wonderland.* It now has a pleasantly old-fashioned air. *See
  also* **Adelaide.**
>   Alecia, Ali, Alicia, Alis, Alisanne, Alisha, Alison,
>   Alissa, Alleece, Allis, Alyce, Alyson, Ellissa

Alida *Lat.* "Small winged one."
>   Alidah, Alita, Allida

Alima *Arab.* "Cultured."

Alina *Slavic.* Variation of **Helen** (*Gk.* "Light").
>   Alena

Alisa *Heb.* "Great happiness."
>   Alisah, Alissa, Aliza

Alison Diminutive of **Alice** (*OG.* "Noble, nobility").
>   Alisanne, Alisoun, Allisann, Allison, Allyson,
>   Alysanne

Alix *OG.* "Noble." *See also* **Alexandra.**
>   Alex

Aliya *Arab.* "Highborn."

    Aaliya, Aaliyah, Alia, Aliyah

Allegra *It.* "Joyous." The musical term *allegro* means "quickly, with a happy air."

    Alegra, Allegretta

Allena (*Fem.* **Alan, Allen**) *Ir. Gael.* Possible meaning "rock" or "comely." *See also* **Alanna.**

    Alana, Alanis, Alene, Alynne

Alma *Lat.* "Giving nurture"; *It.* "Soul"; *Arab.* "Learned." The most common usage, of course, is "alma mater" for a college or university.

Almira (*Fem.* **Elmer**) *Arab.* "Aristocratic lady."

    Almeeria, Almera, Elmera, Elmira, Elmyra

Alona *Heb.* "Oak tree." The many different spellings of this name attest to its use all over Europe.

    Allona, Allonia, Alonia, Elona, Ilona, Ilonka

Althea *Gk.* "With healing power."

    Altheda, Althia

Alva *Sp.* "Blonde, fair-skinned"; *Heb.* "Foliage." *See also* **Albina.**

    Alba, Albina, Albine, Albinia, Alvah

Alvina (*Fem.* **Alvin**) *OE.* "Noble friend" or "elf friend."

    Alvinia, Alwyne, Elvina, Elvinia

Alyssa *Gk.* "Rational." Also the name of a bright yellow flower, alyssum, and its use may have been influenced by the

19th-century vogue for flower names. *See also* the variants of **Alice**.

    Alissa, Allissa, Alysa, Ilyssa, Lyssa

Ama *Ghanaian.* "Born on Saturday."

Amabel *Lat.* "Lovable, amiable." *See also* **Mabel**.

    Amabelle, Belle

Amal *Arab.* "Hope."

    Amahla, Amala

Amanda *Lat.* "Much loved." Regularly used since the 17th century and a top 10 name in the United States from 1976 to 1996. Its use is dwindling now, however.

    Amandine, Manda, Mandee, Mandie

Amara *Gk.* "Lovely forever."

Amber *OF.* Name of the gold-brown semiprecious stone. Jewel names were popular in the 19th century, and Amber came to prominence again in the 1960s. Perhaps because it is a good descriptive name for a golden-skinned baby, Amber is quite well used today.

    Ambar, Amberetta

Amelia *OG.* "Industrious." The 18th-century Princess Amelia brought the name to Britain, where it was popular in the 19th century. *See also* **Emily**.

    Amalia, Amalie, Amalya, Amelie, Ameline, Amilia, Amy, Emelie, Emma, Emmeline, Malia, Malika, Millie, Molly

Amica *Lat.* "Friend." Very unusual. Closely related to Spanish *amiga* or Italian *amica,* the everyday words for "friend" in those languages.

Amilia *Lat.* "Amiable." Also possible variant spelling for **Amelia** or **Emilia.**

　　Amiliya, Amillia

Amina *Arab.* "Honest, trustworthy." Mother of the prophet Muhammad.

　　Ameena, Aminah, Amyna

Amira *Arab.* "Highborn girl."

　　Ameera, Amera, Amirah, Meera, Mira

Amisa *Heb.* "Companion, friend."

　　Amissa

Amita *Heb.* "Truth"; *It.* "Friendship." *See also* **Amica, Amy.**

Amity *Lat.* "Friendship, harmony."

　　Amitie

Amor *Sp.* "Love."

　　Amora, Amore, Amorra

Amorette *Fr.* "Little love."

　　Amoretta

Amy *Lat.* "Loved." In spite of the prominence given the name by Louisa May Alcott's *Little Women,* it didn't become a favorite until the 1950s. Hugely popular in the 1970s, but those women are now becoming mothers and choosing different names.

　　Aimée, Aimie, Amata, Amé, Ami, Amie, Esmé

Anastasia *Gk.* "Resurrection." Indelibly associated with the
daughter of Czar Nicholas II who was rumored to have
escaped death when her family was assassinated during
the Russian Revolution. The name is still something of a
mouthful, but it is much more popular than its short forms
such as **Stacey**.

> Ana, Anastasija, Anastassia, Nastassja, Stacey,
> Stacie, Taisie, Tasha, Tasja, Tasya

Andrea *(Fem. Andrew) Gk.* "A man's woman." Used very
steadily without ever becoming truly fashionable.

> Aindrea, Andee, Andra, Andreana, Andrée,
> Andria, Andy, Ohndrea, Ondrea

Anemone *Gk.* "Breath." In Greek mythology, Anemone was
the name of a nymph who was turned into a flower, which
is also called a windflower.

> Anemona, Anne-Aymone

Angela *Gk.* "Messenger from God, angel." **Angel** was
originally used as a name for men, and in Latin countries
Angelo is still popular. Angela came into frequent use in
the early 20th century.

> Angel, Angele, Angeleta, Angelica, Angelika,
> Angelina, Angeline, Angelique, Angelita, Angelle,
> Angie, Anjela, Anjelika, Gelya

Anisah *Arab.* "Friendly, congenial."

> Anisa, Annissa

Anita *Sp.* form of **Ann.** Most common in the 1950s.

Ann Anglicization of **Hannah** (*Heb.* "Grace"). One of the most
frequently used names for girls until the mid-19th century.
The European form **Anna** is now much more fashionable
(in the top 20) than plain old Ann in the United States, and
Annie is used as often as **Anne**.

> Ana, Anette, Ania, Anissa, Anita, Anitra, Anna,
> Annabel, Annelore, Annick, Annie, Annora,
> Anouk, Anouska, Anya, Hana, Hanna, Hannah,
> Hanni, Nan, Nana, Nance, Nanci, Nancy,
> Nanette, Nannie, Nona, Nonnie

Annabel Possibly a combination of **Anna** and **Belle**: "grace-
ful" and "beautiful." Also mutation of **Amabel**.

> Anabel, Anabella, Annabelinda, Annabelle

Annemarie Combination of **Ann** and **Mary**. The reverse
form, **Marianne**, is also frequently used. The popularity of
the pairing may originate in Roman Catholic veneration of
Saint Anne and Saint Mary, mother and daughter.

> Annamaria

Annette Diminutive of **Ann**. Elaborated forms such as
Annetta may also be considered variations of **Agnes**.

> Anet, Anetta

Annis *Gk.* "Finished, completed." May be easily confused
by the ear with **Agnes**, a point prospective parents might
keep in mind. *See also* variants of **Ann**.

> Anissa, Annes, Annice, Annys

Annora *Lat.* "Honor." A phonetic version of **Honora.**
>   Anora, Honor, Nora, Norah

Annunciata *Lat.* Allusion to the Annunciation, when the
>   Virgin Mary learned she would be the mother of Jesus.
>   Sometimes given to a girl born in March, the logical month
>   for such an announcement.
>   Anonciada, Anunciata, Anunziata

Anonna *Lat.* Name of the Roman goddess of the annual
>   harvest. An appropriate name for an October or November
>   baby.
>   Anona, Nona

Anselma (*Fem.* **Anselm**; *OG.* "Godly helmet") The short
>   forms are much more common.
>   Selma, Zelma

Anthea *Gk.* "Flowerlike." Used by English 17th-century poets
>   to symbolize spring but used infrequently in real life.
>   Antheia, Thia

Anthemia *Gk.* "In bloom." From the same Greek root as
>   **Anthea.**
>   Antheemia, Anthemya, Anthymia

Antoinette (*Fem.* **Anthony**) *Lat.* "Beyond price, invaluable."
>   Also a diminutive of **Ann.** Irresistibly associated with the
>   ill-fated French queen Marie Antoinette.
>   Antonia, Antonie, Antonine, Antwanetta, Netta,
>   Toinette, Toni, Tonia, Tonya

April *Lat.* "Opening up." First used as a name in the 20th century, it occurs most often for a girl born in that month. Curiously, only the months April, **May,** and **June** are used regularly for names, with April the most popular.

    Aprill, Averel, Averell, Avril

Ara *Arab.* "Brings rain."

Arabella *Lat.* "Answered prayer." Unusual name that occurs most frequently in England.

    Arabel, Arbela, Arbella, Bella, Orabel

Arcadia *Gk.* Originally the place name of a region in Greece that eventually came to stand for the home of simple pastoral happiness.

    Arcadie

Arda *Heb.* "Bronze."

    Ardah, Ardath

Arden *Lat.* "Burning with enthusiasm." The Forest of Arden in Shakespeare's *As You Like It* was a magically beautiful place.

    Ardeen, Ardelle, Ardena, Ardin, Ardis

Arella *Heb.* "Messenger from God, angel."

    Arela, Arelle

Aria *It.* "A melody." In the classical operatic form, arias are solos performed by the leading characters.

Ariadne *Gk.* The mythological daughter of the Cretan king Minos, who gave Theseus a thread to guide him out of the mazelike prison known as the Labyrinth.

Ariadna, Ariana, Ariane, Arianna, Aryanna,
Aryanne

Ariana *Welsh.* "Like silver." This is also the Italian version of
Ariadne.

Ariane, Arianna

Ariel *Heb.* "Lioness of God." In Shakespeare's *The Tempest,*
Ariel is a sprite who can disappear at will. The name has
the connotation of something otherworldly, and though
Shakespeare's Ariel is male, the name is used mostly for
girls.

Aeriel, Aeriela, Ariela, Arielle

Arista *Gk.* "The best."

Aristella, Aristelle

Arlene Derivation unclear. Possibly diminutive of **Charles**
(*OE.* "Man") or feminine form of **Arlen** (related to *Gael.*
"Pledge"). The name first appeared in the mid-19th cen-
tury and was popular by the 1930s.

Arla, Arlana, Arleen, Arlen, Arline, Arlyn, Lene

Asención *Sp.* "Ascension," marking Christ's ascension into
heaven, which is commemorated 40 days after Easter.

Asunción

Ashanti *Af.* Area in West Africa from where many American
slaves came. Used in modern American black families.

Ashanta, Ashantae, Ashante, Ashantee,
Ashaunta, Shantee, Shanti, Shauntae

Ashira *Heb.* "Rich" or "I will sing."

> **Asheera, Ashirah**

Ashley *OE.* Place name: "ash tree meadow." Originally a
surname that migrated to first-name status, possibly
helped along by Ashley Wilkes in Margaret Mitchell's *Gone
with the Wind*. Though originally used for boys, it is now
tremendously popular for girls, having been in the top 10
female names since 1982. Only in 2003 did it drop out of
the top 5, a possible sign that it's losing steam.

> **Ashely, Ashlee, Ashleigh, Ashlen, Ashlie**

Asia Name of the continent. The feminine "-ia" ending lends
itself to adaptation as a girl's name.

> **Aja, Asiah, Azha**

Asima *Arab.* "Guardian."

Asta *Gk.* "Like a star." Also short form of **Anastasia, Astrid,**
and **Augusta.** The most famous Asta is probably the ter-
rier owned by Nick and Nora Charles in the famous *Thin
Man* movies of the 1930s.

> **Astera, Asteria, Astra, Estella, Esther, Etoile,
> Hester, Stella**

Astra *Lat.* "Starlike, of the stars." First appeared in the 1940s,
though other star names, such as **Estella,** have been
around longer.

> **Asteria, Asterina, Astria**

Astrid *ONorse.* "Beautiful like a god." Unusual in English-speaking countries, but the name occurs in the royal families of Norway and Belgium.

Astra, Astri, Astride, Astrud

Asunción *Sp.* Marking the Virgin Mary's ascent into heaven, which is commemorated on August 15.

Asención

Atara *Heb.* "Diadem."

Atera, Ateret

Athalia *Heb.* "The Lord is exalted." In the Old Testament, Athalia was the wife of the king of Judah.

Atalee, Atalia, Atalie, Athalie

Athena *Gk.* The goddess of wisdom in Greek mythology. She was a virgin deity who sprang fully armed from Zeus's head. In the *Odyssey,* Homer frequently refers to her as "gray-eyed Athena."

Athenais, Athene, Athina

Atifa *Arab.* "Empathy, affection."

Ateefa, Atifah

Aubrey *OF.* "Elf ruler." Originally a man's name that arrived in England with the Norman Conquest. For a girl, the ear will readily confuse it with the more common **Audrey.**

Aubery, Aubree, Aubreigh, Aubry

Audrey *OE.* "Noble strength." Most popular in the 1920s and 1930s, now less used but still familiar.

Audie, Audra, Audree, Audria, Audrie

Augusta (*Fem.* **Augustus**) *Lat.* "Worthy of respect."
Imported to England by the German mother of George III.
Though common enough in the 18th and 19th centuries, it
is little used now.

> **Auguste, Augustia, Augustina, Augustine,**
> **Austina, Gussie, Tina**

Aura *Gk.* "Soft breeze"; *Lat.* "Gold." Most familiar now, perhaps, in its psychic sense, meaning the atmosphere sur-
rounding an individual.

> **Aure, Aurea, Auria, Oria**

Aurelia *Lat.* "Gold." Originally a name used by Roman clans,
it resurfaced as a first name in the 19th century.

> **Auralia, Aurea, Aurel, Aurélie, Aurelina, Oralia**

Aurora *Lat.* "Dawn." Aurora was the Roman goddess of
sunrise. Used by 19th-century poets such as Byron and
Browning, but never common.

> **Aurore, Ora**

Austine (*Fem.* **Augustine** or **Austin**) *Lat.* "Worthy of respect."

Autumn Season name, only recently used as a first name.

Ava *Lat.* "Like a bird." May have originated as a form of **Eva.**

Avalon *Celt.* "Island of apples." In Celtic myth, Avalon is an
island paradise. In Arthurian legend, it is the island where
King Arthur took refuge after his final defeat and whence
he will reappear.

Aviva *Heb.* "Springlike, fresh, dewy."

    Avivah

Avril A French version of **April,** the month name. Also possibly a version of the name of a 7th-century saint, Everild.

    Averel, Averill

Aya *Heb.* "Bird."

    Ayla

Ayanna Recently invented name that may be considered an elaboration of **Anna** or of the typically feminine "-ana" ending. Probably popular because it sounds pretty.

    Aiyana, Aiyanna, Ayana, Iana, Ianna

Ayesha *Per.* "Small one."

Aza *Arab.* "Comfort."

Azelia *Heb.* "Aided by God."

Aziza *Heb.* "Mighty"; *Arab.* "Precious."

Azura *OF.* "Azure, sky blue." A good attribute name for a blue-eyed baby.

    Azora, Azure, Azzura

Babe Diminutive of **Barbara** (*Gk.* "Foreign"). Also short for "baby," as in "See ya, babe."

Babette *Fr.* Diminutive of **Barbara** (*Gk.* "Foreign").

Bailey *OE.* "Law enforcer, bailiff." A surname that metamorphosed into a first name in the 19th century, now substantially used for girls.

> **Bailee, Baily**

Baptista *Lat.* "One who baptizes."

> **Baptiste, Battista, Bautista**

Bara *Heb.* "To select."

> **Barah, Bari, Barra, Barrie**

Barbara *Gk.* "Foreign." The adjective was originally applied to anyone who did not speak Greek; it has the same root as "barbarian." The early Christian martyr Saint Barbara was imprisoned in a tower by her father; she is patroness of engineers and architects. The name had its greatest popularity in the 19th to 20th centuries, peaking around 1925, when in the United States it was second only to **Mary.**

> **Baba, Babara, Babe, Babette, Babs, Barbary, Barbie, Barbra, Basia, Bobbi, Bobbie, Bonnie, Bonny, Varvara, Varina**

Bathsheba *Heb.* "Daughter of the oath." Biblical name: Bathsheba was the mistress and later the wife of King David. Surprisingly (given her history), the name was used often by the Puritans.

> **Bathseva, Bathshua, Batsheba, Batya, Bethsabée, Sheba, Sheva**

Batya *Heb.* "God's daughter."

> **Bitya, Basha**

Beata *Lat.* "Blessed." First word of the Latin version of the
famous beatitudes section of the biblical Sermon on the
Mount: "Blessed are the poor in spirit." A popular name in
northern Europe.
> **Bea, Beate**

Beatrice *Lat.* "Bringer of gladness." The original form,
Beatrix, was often found in the Middle Ages in England,
then forgotten until its Victorian revival as Beatrice. It fell
out of fashion after the 1920s and is very rare today.
> **Bea, Beatrix, Bebe, Bee, Trixie, Trixy**

Bebba *Heb.* "God's pledge."

Becky Diminutive of **Rebecca** (*Heb.* "Noose"). Occasionally
used as an independent first name.

Behira *Heb.* "Shining, bright."

Belinda Unclear origin; possibly combination of **Belle** and
Linda.
> **Bellinda, Belynda, Linda**

Belita *Sp.* "Little beauty."
> **Bellita**

Bell Diminutive of **Isabel** (*Heb.* "Pledged to God"). Also, surname used as a first name.

Bella *Lat.* "Beautiful." Or diminutive of **Isabella** (*Heb.*
"Pledged to God"). Used as early as the Middle Ages, but it
was not popular until the 18th century.
> **Bell, Belle**

Belle *Fr.* "Beautiful." Enjoyed a brief fad in the 1870s but almost unheard of since then.

>   Belinda, Bella

Benita *Sp.* Variant of **Benedicta.** More common than Benedicta but very unusual in English-speaking countries.

>   Benedetta, Benedicta, Bénédicte, Benedikta, Benetta, Bennie, Benôite

Bentley *OE.* "Meadow of ben (grass)." Place name that became surname, then first name, but scarce. Linked in most minds with the luxurious English cars.

>   Bentlea, Bentlee, Bentleigh

Bernadette (*Fem.* **Bernard.**) *Fr.* "Bear/courageous." Made famous by Saint Bernadette of Lourdes, a miller's daughter who in 1858 repeatedly saw visions of the Virgin Mary. By the time she was canonized in 1933, Lourdes had become a world-famous destination for pilgrims. The name is now unusual in English-speaking countries.

>   Bennie, Benny, Berna, Bernadetta, Bernadine, Bernie

Bernice *Gk.* "She who brings victory." From the same root as **Veronica.** The name appears in the New Testament and first occurred in Britain in the 16th century, but its only real popularity came at the end of the 19th century. Little used today.

>   Beranice, Berenice, Berenyce, Bernyce, Nixie

Bertha *OG.* "Bright." Also related to the name of a Teutonic goddess. Very popular in the late 19th century but almost unheard of since 1920. This disuse may be explained by the fact that a German cannon used in World War I was nicknamed "Big Bertha" after Bertha Krupp, daughter of the family who manufactured the weapon.

> Berrta, Berta, Berte, Berthe, Birdie, Birta

Beryl *Gk.* "Pale green gemstone." Beryl was considered a to- ken of good luck. The name first appeared with the fashion for jewel names in the late 19th century.

> Berri, Berrie, Beryn

Beth *Heb.* "House." Diminutive of **Elizabeth** (*Heb.* "Pledged to God"), **Bethany**.

Bethany Biblical: the name of the village near Jerusalem where Lazarus lived with his sisters, Mary and Martha. In some cases, a variant on the combined form **Beth-Ann**.

> Bethanee, Bethaney, Bethanie, Bethanne, Bethannie

Bethia *Heb.* "Daughter of Jehovah." Popular in the eras, such as the 17th century, when Old Testament names were intensively used.

> Betia, Bithia

Betty Diminutive of **Elizabeth** (*Heb.* "Pledged to God"). A nickname with great popularity in its own right. It first became common in the 18th century, and after a spell of disuse, it was one of the top names in every

English-speaking country by the 1920s. Now it seems like a period artifact.

Bett, Betta, Bette, Bettie, Bettina

Beulah *Heb.* "Married." Also used to refer to Israel, and in John Bunyan's *The Pilgrim's Progress,* Beulah is the promised land. It first became a girl's name in the late 16th century. References to "Beulah land" appear in American spirituals.

Beula, Bewlah

Beverly *OE.* Place name: "beaver stream." Originally an English place name and a surname, then used for both sexes as a first name. Probably still most famous as a place name, referring to Beverly Hills.

Beverlee, Beverley, Beverlie, Bevlyn

Bianca *It.* "White." The meek younger daughter in Shakespeare's *The Taming of the Shrew* and the subject of a song in the spin-off musical *Kiss Me, Kate.*

Biancha, Blanca

Bibi *Arab.* "Lady."

Bebe

Bibiana *Sp.* Variation of **Vivian** (*Lat.* "Alive").

Bibiane, Bibianna

Billie *OE.* Diminutive of **Wilhelmina** (*OG.* "Will helmet"). Feminine use of what is generally considered a man's name; more popular in the South, though uncommon now.

Billa, Billee, Willa

Blaine *Ir. Gael.* "Slender." Surname now used as a first name, more common for boys. Cropped up as a first name in the 1930s.

> **Blane, Blayne**

Blair *Scot. Gael.* Place name referring to a plain or flat area. Surname now used as a first name, though scarce.

> **Blaire**

Blanche *Fr.* "White, pale." Very popular in the United States at the end of the 19th century but unusual now.

> **Bellanca, Bianca, Blanca**

Blanchefleur *Fr.* "White flower."

Blessing *OE.* "Consecration."

Blimah *Heb.* "Blossom."

> **Blima, Blime**

Bliss *OE.* "Intense happiness." Least common of the "happiness" names: **Allegria, Felicia, Hillary, Joy.**

> **Blisse, Blyss**

Blossom *OE.* "Flowerlike." Generic flower name used mostly at the turn of the 20th century.

Blythe *OE.* "Happy, carefree." Made famous by the opening lines of Shelley's poem "To a Skylark" ("Hail to thee, blithe spirit!") and Noel Coward's play *Blithe Spirit.*

> **Blithe**

Bobbie Diminutive of **Roberta** (*OE.* "Bright renown"). Like **Billie**, a feminine version of a man's nickname. Also derives from **Barbara** (*Gk.* "Stranger").

Bonita *Sp.* "Pretty." Popular in the early 1940s but unusual now.

Bonnie *Scot.* "Good, fair of face." The Scots adopted the French word *bonne,* meaning "good." An old nursery rhyme claims, "The child who is born on the Sabbath Day/ Is bonny and blithe and good and gay," which makes this an appropriate name for Sunday's child.

> Bonne, Bonnebell, Bonnee

Brandy Name of a liquor. In the early 1980s, one of the most popular names for American girls, reaching the top 10 in some surveys. Like most trendy names, it has lost favor rather rapidly.

> Brandais, Brandea, Brandee, Brandi, Brandice, Brandie

Brenda (*Fem.* **Brendan**) *OE.* "Burning." One source translates the Irish as "stinking hair," though the origin may also be a Norse word for "sword." Brenda was originally a Scottish name and was particularly fashionable in the 1940s.

> Brenn, Brennda

Brenna *Ir. Gael.* "Raven; black-haired." Also diminutive of **Brendan.**

> Bren, Brennah, Brinna

Brett *Lat.* "From Britain." Surname transferred to first name. Still more common for boys.

> Brette, Britt

Brianna (*Fem.* **Brian**) *Ir. Gael.* Meaning obscure, possibly "strong" or "hill." In the top 20 names since the mid-1990s, probably because of its pleasant sound.

> Breana, Breanne, Bria, Briana, Brinna, Bryana, Bryanne, Bryn, Brynne

Bridget *Ir. Gael.* "Strength, power." May also derive from the name of a goddess of ancient Ireland. Very popular name in Ireland from the 18th century to the 1950s—so much so that in the late 19th century in the United States the stock figure of the Irish housemaid (in plays, cartoons, etc.) was frequently called Bridget.

> Beret, Berget, Biddie, Birget, Birgit, Birgitta, Breeda, Bride, Bridey, Bridgett, Bridgit, Bridie, Brighid, Brigid, Brigidine, Brigit, Brigitte, Brita, Britt, Britte, Brydie, Brygid

Brie *Fr.* Place name for a region in France most famous for the production of its cheese.

> Bree, Briette

Brier *Fr.* "Heather." Unusual botanical name. Though the personal name derives from the French term for heather, the word in English usually describes a wild rose with small, prickly thorns. In some versions of *Sleeping Beauty,* Prince Charming has to cut through a hedge of briars to reach the princess.

> Briar

Brittany *Lat.* "From England." According to records kept by the U.S. government, this was the sixth most popular girl's name in the 1990s, though it has been sliding down the lists since 1990.

> Briteny, Britney, Britni, Britt, Brittan, Brittaney, Britteny

Brooke *OE.* Place name: "small stream." Also a surname and originally more common for boys. Now clearly a feminine name.

> Brook, Brookie, Brooks

Brunhilda *OG.* "Armor-wearing fighting maid." Heroine of the Siegfried legend popularized in the *Ring* cycle of operas by Richard Wagner. Brunhilda is one of the Valkyrie—maidens who ride into battle.

> Brinhild, Brinhilda, Brinhilde, Brunhild, Brunhilde, Brynhilda, Brynhilde, Hilda

Bryn *Welsh.* "Mount." Another place name converted to a Christian name in the 20th century.

> Brinna, Brynn, Brynne

Caitlin *Ir.* Along with **Megan,** Caitlin has been very popular recently among families with no Irish ties whatsoever. *See also* **Catherine.**

  Caitlan, Caitlyn, Catelynn, Caylin, Kaitlynn, Katelin

Calla *Gk.* "Beautiful." Also the name of a flower, though the calla lily, with its smooth, sculptured lines, was not fashionable at the same time as the general vogue for flower names.

Calliope *Gk.* Muse of epic poetry. Also the name of a musical instrument typically seen at circuses and carnivals. *See also* **Clio.**

  Callia, Kalliope

Callista *Gk.* "Most beautiful."

  Cala, Calesta, Calista, Kalista

Calypso *Gk.* "She who hides." In Greek mythology the nymph Calypso held Odysseus captive on an island for seven years. The name is also applied to the lilting music of the West Indies.

  Calipso, Callypso, Kallypso

Camellia Flower name first used in the 1930s when the rather exotic blooms were quite fashionable. Its root is actually distinct from the more common **Camille.**

Camelia, Cammelia, Kamelia

Cameo *It. from Middle French.* "Skin." A stone or shell (frequently pinkish) carved with a picture, often a tiny portrait. Cameos have been very popular as jewelry at various periods, most recently the Victorian era.

Cammeo

Cameron *Scot. Gael.* "Crooked nose." Clan name derived from the facial feature. Little used as a first name, even for boys, until the middle of the 20th century.

Camron, Camryn, Kameron

Camilla *Lat.* Meaning unclear, though some sources trace it to the young girls who assisted at pagan religious ceremonies. The name has been used consistently since the 19th century.

Cama, Camila, Camille, Cammie, Kamila, Milla, Millie, Milly

Candace Possibly *Lat.* "Brilliantly white." Historically the name was the ancient title of the queens of Ethiopia before the 4th century. Not much used until the mid-20th century.

Candaice, Candayce, Candee, Candie, Candiss, Candyce, Dacie, Dacy, Kandace

Candida *Lat.* "White." Popular in the early Christian era, then very rare until the 20th century, when it has been used occasionally.

Candi, Candide

Cara *Lat.* "Darling." Began to be fashionable from the 1970s onward.

> Caralie, Caretta, Carina, Carine, Carrie, Kara, Karina

Carey *Welsh.* Place name: "near the castle." A name used for both men and women. In this form it is a transferred surname, but it may be considered a diminutive of **Caroline**, especially for women.

> Carrey, Cary

Carissa *Gk.* "Grace." Also possibly another variation of **Cara**. *See also* **Charis**.

> Caresa, Caressa, Charissa, Karisa

Carita *Lat.* "Beloved." Also possibly derived from the Latin word for charity, *caritas.*

Carla (*Fem. Carl*) Diminutive of **Caroline** (*OG.* "Man"). A European-sounding version of the many names that derive from **Charles**.

> Carlana, Carlette, Carlla, Karla

Carlin *Gael.* "Little champion."

> Carling

Carly (*Fem. Charles*) Diminutive of **Caroline, Charlotte** (*OG.* "Man"). The form **Carleen** (or **Carlene**) was primarily a product of the 1960s; this shorter version is now more popular.

> Carleen, Carlene, Carley, Carline, Carly, Karlie

Carmel *Heb.* "Garden." Biblical place name: Mount Carmel is in Israel and is often referred to as a kind of paradise. The name has been used by Catholic families for some hundred years, though the form **Carmen** is much more common.

> Carma, Carmela, Carmelina, Carmelit, Carmelita, Carmiela, Carmine, Carmy, Karmel, Karmen

Carmen *Lat.* "Song." Also a derivation of **Carmel.** One of the titles of the Virgin Mary is Santa Maria del Carmen (meaning Saint Mary of Mount Carmel), and this form of the name honors her.

> Carmencita, Carmie, Carmina, Carmine, Carmita

Carol (*Fem.* **Carl, Charles**) *OG.* "Man." Originally a short form of **Caroline,** not an adoption of "Christmas carol." It first appeared about a hundred years ago, and it was enormously popular by the mid-20th century. The popularity of the name peaked in the mid-sixties, and it is now out of style.

> Carel, Carey, Caro, Carola, Carole, Caroll, Caroly, Carroll, Caryl, Caryll, Karel, Kari, Karole

Caroline (*Fem.* **Carl, Charles**) *OG.* "Man." A rather stately diminutive with royal connotations. The name was brought to England by George II's queen and was popular until the end of the 19th century. It is now enjoying a mild revival.

> Caraleen, Caraline, Caralyn, Caralynn, Carla,

Carlene, Carley, Carlin, Carlina, Carlita, Carlota,
Carlotta, Carly, Carlyn, Carlyna, Carlyne, Carlynn,
Carlynne, Carol, Carola, Carole, Carolin, Carolina,
Carolyne, Carrie, Carollyn, Cary, Charline,
Karalyn, Karoline, Lina, Sharla, Sharline

Casey *Ir. Gael.* "Watchful." Used for both boys and girls.

Cacie, Caisie, Caycey, Kacey, Kayci, Kaysey

Cassandra *Gk.* Perhaps a version of **Alexander.** In Greek
mythology, she was the daughter of King Priam of Troy.

Casandera, Cassandre, Cassaundra, Kassandra,
Sondra, Zandra

Cassidy *Ir.* "Clever." Surname transferred to male first name
transferred to girl's name.

Cassady, Cassidey, Kassadey

Catherine *Gk.* "Pure." One of the oldest recorded names,
with roots in Greek antiquity. Almost every Western country
has its own form of the name, and phonetic variations are
endless. Though not trendy, it is very frequently used, especially if you take alternative spellings such as **Katherine**
and **Kathryn** into account.

Cait, Caitlin, Caitrionagh, Caren, Cari, Caronne,
Cass, Cataleena, Catalina, Catarine, Cate,
Cathaleen, Catharine, Cathe, Cathelle, Catheryn,
Cathie, Cathrynn, Cathy, Catina, Catrionagh,
Cazzy, Ekaterina, Karen, Kasja, Kaska, Katalin,
Katelle, Katha, Katherin, Kathleen, Kathy,

> Katinka, Katlaina, Katushka, Katya, Kay, Kit, Kitty, Trina, Yekaterina

Cecilia (*Fem.* **Cecil**) *Lat.* "Blind one." From a Roman clan name. Saint Cecilia is the patroness of music. The name was used in Roman times, then resurfaced in the Victorian era. The form **Cecily** was briefly popular in the 1920s, but neither name has been used much since then.

> Ceceley, Cecil, Cecile, Ceciliane, Cecilija, Cecilla, Cecily, Cecilyann, Ceil, Cela, Celia, Celie, Cesya, Cicely, Cile, Cilia, Cilka, Cilla, Cissie, Seely, Seelya, Sesilia, Sessile, Sissy

Celena *Gk.* Goddess of the moon, later identified with Artemis. A version of the more common **Selina**, although neither name is frequently used.

> Cela, Celina

Celeste *Lat.* "Heavenly." Unusual in any of its forms. Parents may associate the name with Queen Celeste, wife of the children's book character Babar, the elephant.

> Cela, Celesta, Celestia, Celestina, Celestine, Celina, Celinda, Celine, Celleste, Selestia

Chanah *Heb.* "Grace." *See also* **Hannah**.

> Chana, Chanach

Chandra *Sanskrit.* "Like the moon." The greatest Hindu goddess Devi is also known as Chandra.

> Chandi, Shandra

Chanel *Fr.* Surname of the legendary fashion designer Coco
   Chanel, and by extension, the name of a number of famous perfumes. Began to be used as a first name in the
   1980s.
   Chanelle, Shanelle

Chantal *Fr.* Originally a place name meaning "stony spot,"
   but possibly also derived from the verb *chanter*, "to sing."
   Unusual in the United States.
   Chantalle, Chantelle, Shantalle, Shontelle

Charis *Gk.* "Grace." One of the mythological Three Graces.
   Charisse, Charys, Karis

Charity *Lat.* "Brotherly love." One of the three cardinal
   virtues, along with Faith and Hope. They have survived
   better than many of the other virtue names (Temperance,
   Fortitude, Humility, Chastity, Mercy, Obedience) popular
   among the Puritans in the 17th century.
   Carissa, Carita, Charita, Charitey, Chariza

Charlotte *Fr.* "Little and womanly." One of the most popular
   feminine forms of **Charles**. Like **Caroline**, Charlotte was
   popularized in England by a queen (George III's wife) and
   was much used from the 18th century to the beginning of
   the 20th. With the recent return to old-fashioned names, it
   has been dusted off for a reappearance.
   **Carlotta, Carly, Charlaine, Charmion, Charty,
   Karlota, Karlyne, Lola, Lottie, Sharlot, Sharyl**

Charmaine From a Latin clan name; also possibly related to **Carmen** and **Caroline.** Enjoyed bursts of popularity in the 1920s and 1950s.

Charmain, Charmayne, Sharmain

Charmian *Gk.* "Joy." A distinctly separate name from **Charmaine,** though they are often confused. Because of its Greek origin, Charmian should be pronounced with a hard C, but it rarely is.

Charmiane, Charmyan

Chasidah *Heb.* "Devout woman."

Chava *Heb.* "Life."

Chaya, Eva, Hava

Chaviva *Heb.* "Beloved."

Eva

Chelsea *OE.* "Port or landing place." Place name; possibly owes some of its appeal to British pop culture of the late 1960s.

Chelcie, Chelseigh, Chelsey

Cher *Fr.* "Beloved." For most people, inseparable from the singer and actress who uses this name alone without a surname. Somewhat popular in the late 1960s and early 1970s.

Chere, Cherée, Cheri, Cherie

Cheryl Familiar form of **Charlotte.** A 20th-century name that first became popular in the 1940s and increased in use

into the 1960s. Like most 60-year-old fashions, it is now
quite dated.

    Charil, Charyl, Cherilyn, Cherryl, Cheryll, Sharyl,
    Sheril, Sherill, Sheryl

Chiara *It.* "Light." *See also* **Claire.**

    Chiarra, Kiara

Chloe *Gk.* "Young green shoot." Appears in the Bible and as a
name in literature. Since 2000, it has become increasingly
popular in the United States.

    Clo, Cloe, Cloey

Christabel *Lat./Fr.* "Fair Christian." Use has been primarily
literary.

    Christabella, Christabelle, Christobel, Cristabel

Christina (*Fem. Christian*) *Gk.* "Anointed, Christian."
Christian was used for women in medieval times. By the
18th century, Christina was the more common form. It was
superseded in the 1930s by the French form **Christine.**
The cycle of fashion has now brought Christina back to
solid but not trendy popularity.

    Chris, Chrissie, Chrissy, Christan, Christel,
    Christiana, Christiane, Christy, Chrystalle,
    Crissie, Cristen, Cristina, Khristina, Kirstin, Kris,
    Kristina, Krysta, Tina

Chumani *Sioux.* "Drops of dew."

Cindy Originally a nickname for **Cynthia** (*Gk.* "Goddess from

Mt. Cynthos") or **Lucinda** (*Lat.* "Light"). Popular for children born in the fifties and sixties.

> Cindee, Cindi, Cindie, Cyndie, Cyndy, Sindee

Claire *Lat.* "Bright." The original form was **Clare,** as in Saint Clare, the 13th-century founder of a Franciscan order of nuns. In the 19th century, **Clara** became fashionable, but since the 1960s, the French form Claire has dominated.

> Chiara, Ciara, Clairene, Clairette, Clarabel, Clarice, Clarine, Clarissa, Clary, Clorinda, Klara

Clara *Lat.* "Bright." Another version of **Claire,** but one that has been very rare for some time.

> Clarabelle, Claribel, Clarice, Clarinda, Clarita, Klara

Clarice Variant of **Claire** that enjoyed a flurry of popularity around the turn of the 20th century. **Clarissa** is a Latinized version.

> Clarissa, Clarisse, Claryce, Klarissa

Claudia (*Fem.* **Claude, Claudius**) *Lat.* Clan name probably meaning "lame."

> Claude, Claudella, Claudelle, Claudette, Claudina, Claudine

Clea Unknown derivation, but possibly invented by author Lawrence Durrell for a character in his famous Alexandria Quartet.

Clementine *Lat.* "Mild, giving mercy."
> Clemence, Clemency, Clementia, Clementina,
> Clementya

Clio *Gk.* Muse of history.

Clorinda *Lat.* Literary name coined by 16th-century Italian poet Tasso.

Clover *OE.* Flower name. Perhaps because of the modest nature of the flower, the name occurred in the 19th century more commonly as a nickname.

Colette Diminutive of **Nicole** (*Gk./Fr.* "People of victory"). Used mostly since the 1940s, though never widespread.
> Coletta, Collette, Nicolette

Colleen *Ir. Gael.* "Girl." In use since the 1940s in English-speaking countries *except* Ireland.
> Coleen, Collie

Columbine *Lat.* "Dove." Columbine is also a literary character who appears in traditional Italian comedy and English pantomime as Harlequin's beloved. Also a flower name for a delicate two-colored blossom.
> Collie, Columba

Concepción *Lat.* "Conception." Used mostly in Latin American countries to honor the Immaculate Conception and, by extension, the Virgin Mary.
> Cetta, Concetta, Concha, Concheta, Conchita

Constance *Lat.* "Steadfastness." Used often in the early Christian and medieval eras, then by the Puritans. Revived briefly in the early 1900s.

>Con, Connie, Conny, Constancia, Costanza, Konstance

Consuelo *Sp.* "Consolation, comfort." Honors Santa Maria del Consuelo.

>Consolata, Consuela

Cora *Gk.* "Maiden." Though some sources trace the name to classical mythology, its modern form was probably coined by American writer James Fenimore Cooper in *The Last of the Mohicans* (1826).

>Corabelle, Corella, Coretta, Corey, Corinna, Corinne, Corisande, Corrissa, Korella

Coral *Lat.* Nature name: first appeared during the Victorian vogue for jewel names, usually in England.

>Coralee, Coralena, Coralie, Coraline, Koralie

Corazón *Sp.* "Heart."

Cordelia Derivation unclear but probably related to Latin *cor* or "heart."

>Cordelie, Cordella, Cordelle, Cordy, Delia, Delie, Della, Kordelia

Corey *Ir. Gael.* Place name: "the hollow." Place name transferred to surname.

>Corrie, Korry

Corinne French form of **Cora,** used since the 1860s.

> Corina, Corinda, Corine, Corinna, Corrienne,
> Corrinda

Cornelia (*Fem.* **Cornelius**) *Lat.* "Like a horn." Comes from a famous Latin clan name.

> Cornalia, Cornela, Cornelija

Cosima (*Fem.* **Cosmo**) *Gk.* "Order." Very unusual in English-speaking countries.

> Cosma, Cosmé, Kosma

Courtney *OE.* "Court dweller." Surname transferred to first name; usually feminine in the United States. Immensely popular in the 1990s.

> Cortenay, Corteney, Cortnee, Cortneigh, Cortney,
> Courtenay, Courteneigh, Courteney, Courtnay,
> Kortney

Cressida *Gk.* Heroine of a tale (*Troilus and Cressida*) that has been told by Boccaccio, Chaucer, and Shakespeare.

Cristina *Lat.* "Anointed, Christian." *See also* **Christina.**

Crystal *Gk.* "Ice." Transferred use of the word, mostly modern, and increasing since the 1950s. Curiously enough, Crystal was considered a man's name in Scotland hundreds of years ago, where it was a diminutive of **Christopher.** *See also* **Christina.**

> Christal, Christalle, Chrystal, Chrystalle,
> Chrystel, Cristel, Krystle

Cynthia *Gk.* "Goddess from Mount Cynthos"—that is, Artemis, the moon goddess, who was supposed to have been born there. The name was popular from the 1920s to the 1950s, then was replaced by its nickname, **Cindy,** which is now rare. Many of the diminutives are also variants of **Lucinda.**

> Cinda, Cindee, Cinnie, Cintia, Cinzia, Cynthea, Cynthie, Kynthia, Sindee, Synthya

Cyra (*Fem.* **Cyrus**) *Per.* "Sun" or "throne."

D

Dagmar *OG.* Meaning unclear, though possibly "day's glory." In Denmark, Dagmar is a royal name.

Dahlia *Scan.* Flower name of fairly recent vintage, first used in numbers in the 1920s. The flower itself was named in honor of the 18th-century Swedish botanist Anders Dahl.

> Daleia, Dalia, Dalla

Dai *Jap.* "Great."

Daisy *OE.* "Eye of the day." One of the most popular of the 19th-century flower names. It was often used as a nickname for **Margaret,** since in France the flower is called a *marguerite.* This is the kind of name that nostalgia may resurrect.

Daisee, Daisey

Dale *OE.* Place name: "valley." Originally a surname meaning "one who lives in the valley." The term *dale* is still used in parts of England. Most popular as a first name in the 1930s.

Dayle

Dalila *Swahili.* "Delicate."

Damaris *Gk.* "Calf" is the most commonly proposed meaning, though another source suggests "to tame." A Damaris in the New Testament was converted by Saint Paul, and the Puritans adopted the name with enthusiasm.

Damara, Damaress, Dameris, Demarest, Demaris

Damia *Gk.* Meaning not clear; possibly "to tame," although the Greek root is also close to the word for "spirit." The masculine form, **Damian,** is more often seen.

Damiana, Damiane, Damienne, Damyan

Dana *OE.* "From Denmark." Also a surname, used as a boy's first name in the 19th century, but now almost exclusively a girl's name, specifically an American one.

Danaca, Danay, Dane, Danette, Dania, Danica, Danna, Donnica

Danielle (*Fem.* Daniel) *Heb.* "God is my judge." Uncommon until the middle of the 20th century, when, following a revival of Daniel, it became more fashionable.

Danee, Danele, Danella, Danelle, Danette, Dani,

Dania, Danica, Danice, Daniela, Daniella, Danila, Dannielle

Daphne *Gk.* "Laurel tree." In Greek mythology Daphne was a nymph who, attempting to flee an amorous Apollo, was turned into a laurel tree. The name enjoyed a brief English vogue between 1900 and 1930.

Dafna, Dafne, Daphna

Dara *Heb.* "Nugget of wisdom." In the New Testament, a man's name, but its occasional modern use is for girls. Its resemblance to the familiar **Sarah** and **Tara** probably works in its favor.

Darragh, Darrah

Darcie *Ir. Gael.* "Dark." Also Norman place name: "from Arcy." In Britain, usually a boy's name, but in the United States, it is more likely to be feminine.

D'Arcy, Darcee, Darcey, Darcy

Daria (*Fem.* Darius) *Gk.* "Rich."

Dari, Darian, Darya

Darlene Modern adaptation of "darling" used for a given name. First used in the late 1930s and extremely fashionable by the 1950s in the United States. Now out of style.

Darelle, Darla, Darleen, Darline

Daryl Transferred surname, possibly originated as a French place name, like **Darcy**.

Darrell, Darrelle, Darryl, Darrylene, Darryll, Daryline

Davina (*Fem.* **David**) *Heb.* "Loved one." The most commonly used feminine variant of the hugely popular masculine name.

> Daveen, Daviana, Daviane, Davida, Davidina, Davine, Davinia

Dawn *OE.* "Dawn." Modern use of the word for a name. **Aurora,** the Latin term, dates back some fifteen hundred years, but Dawn first appeared in the late 1920s.

> Dawna, Dawnita, Dawnyelle, Dwan

Daya *Heb.* "Bird of prey."

Dea *Lat.* "Goddess."

Deanna *OE.* Place name: "valley"; occupational name: "church leader." Feminine of **Dean,** which only came into use as a first name in the 1950s. Could also be considered a version of **Diana.**

> Deana, Deanne

Deborah *Heb.* "Bee." One of the few significant women's names to figure in the Old Testament; in the Book of Judges, she was an important prophetess and judge. Predictably, the Puritans latched on to the name, but it was not widely used until the 1950s.

> Deb, Debbee, Debbey, Debbi, Debbie, Debbra, Debby, Deberah, Debi, Debora, Debra, Debrah, Devora, Devorah

Dee *Welsh.* "Swarthy." Diminutive of **Deirdre, Delia,** and **Diana.**

> Dede, Dedie, DeeDee, Didi

Deirdre *Ir.* Possible meanings are "fear" and "raging woman." In Irish mythology, Deirdre was the most beautiful woman in Ireland, whose tragically complex love life caused several deaths, including her own. The name has only been in use since the 1920s.

> Dede, Dedra, Dee, DeeDee, Deidra, Deidre, Deidrie

Delaney *Ir. Gael.* "Offspring of the challenger."

> Delaine, Delainey, Delainy, Delanie, Delany

Delia *Gk.* "From Delos." In Greek mythology, the goddess Artemis was born in Delos, so Delia could be an allusion to her.

> Deelia, Delya

Delight *OF.* The emotion as a name. Scarce.

Delilah *Heb.* "Lovelorn, seductive." In the Old Testament, mistress of Samson. The familiar story of how she cuts off his hair to sap his strength probably limits use of her name.

> Dalila, Delila, Lila, Lilah

Della Short for **Adelaide, Adeline, Adelle.** Used as an independent name since the 1870s.

> Delle

Delphine *Gk.* "Dolphin." This is a French form of a name with a complex origin. It alludes to the Greek town of Delphi, home of a famous oracle. The Greeks believed that Delphi was the earth's womb; the dolphin's shape resembles that of a pregnant woman.

Delfa, Delfine, Delfyne, Delphina, Delphinia

Demetria *Gk.* In Greek mythology, Demeter was goddess
of corn and mother of Persephone, whose abduction to
Hades led to the cycle of seasons.

Demeter, Demetra, Demetria, Demetris

Dena *OE.* Place name: "valley." Use of Dena followed the
popularity of **Dean** in the 1950s.

Deana, Deena, Dina

Denise (*Fem.* **Dennis**) *Fr.* "Follower of Dionysius." Though
there is an ancient Latin form of the name (**Dionysia**),
this variation dates back only to the 1920s. It was very
popular in the 1950s, but since the mid-1960s it has been
eclipsed.

Denice, Deniece, Denisse, Denyce, Denys,
Denyse

Desirée *Fr.* "Much desired." The Puritans used **Desire** as a
given name, though its connotations in the 17th century
were religious rather than erotic. The French form is more
usual today.

Desarae, Deseray, Desir, Desirae, Desiray,
Desirea

Devon *OE.* Place name: a county in southern England. More
common for girls than for boys. **Devin** may also be considered a variant.

Devan, Deven, Devenne

Diamond Unusual jewel name first used in the 1890s. The gem is the birthstone for April.

Diamanta, Diamante

Diana "Divine." The Roman goddess of the moon, corresponding to the Greek Artemis. Used steadily since the 16th century, though the French version **Diane** eclipsed it in the mid-20th century. The apotheosis of Lady Diana Spencer as princess of Wales in 1980 gave Diana new charm for prospective parents, especially in Britain.

Dayanna, Dayanne, Deana, DeeDee, Di, Diahann, Diahanne, Diandra, Diane, Diann, Dianna, Dianne, Dyan, Dyana

Dido *Gk.* In Virgil's *Aeneid,* the queen of Carthage who falls in love with Aeneas and commits suicide when he leaves her. The name's origins are obscure: Virgil may have coined it.

Dilys *Welsh.* "Reliable." Dates from the mid-19th century.

Dillys, Dyllis

Dinah *Heb.* "Justified." Old Testament name. In the United States, it has been popular in the South.

Dina, Dyna, Dynah

Dionne Two possible sources: Dionne is the mother of Aphrodite in Greek mythology. The name can also be a feminine version of **Dion** (*Gk.* "Follower of Dionysus"). It is also a homonym for the French pronunciation of **Diane.**

Deiondra, Deonne, Dion, Diona, Diondra, Dione, Dionna

Dodie *Heb.* "Well loved." Familiar form of **Dora, Dorothy** (*Gk.* "Gift of God").

>   Doda, Dodee, Dodi, Dody

Dolly Familiar form of **Dorothy.** As an independent name, it was most popular at the turn of the 20th century but never a favorite.

>   Dolley, Dollie

Dolores *Sp.* "Sorrows." An allusion to the Virgin Mary, Santa Maria de los Dolores.

>   Delora, Delores, Dolorcitas

Dominique (*Fem.* **Dominic**) *Lat.* "Lord." French form of a Latin name, rather fashionable since the 1980s. Could be used for a child born on Sunday, "the Lord's day."

>   Domenica, Domenique, Dominga, Dominica, Dominika

Donna *It.* "Lady." The original meaning is closer to "lady of the home." Strictly modern use as a given name, dating from the 1920s.

>   Dona, Donelle, Donetta, Donica, Ladonna

Dora *Gk.* "Gift." Probably originated as a diminutive of names such as **Theodora** and introduced as an independent name by a character in Charles Dickens's *David Copperfield.* Its heyday in the United States came at the end of the 19th century.

>   Dodi, Dodie, Doralee, Doralia, Doralina, Dore, Doree, Doreen, Dorie

Dorcas *Gk.* "Gazelle." New Testament name, Greek version of
   Tabitha. Saint Peter raised her from the dead.

Dorée *Fr.* "Gilded."
   Dorae, Doraie, D'Oray, Dore

Doreen Several possible origins, including *Ir. Gael.*
   "Brooding," *Fr.* "Gilded," and an elaboration of **Dora.** In the
   top 10 in Britain in the 1920s, now unusual.
   Dorene, Dorine, Doryne

Doretta *Gk.* "Gift from God." Variant of **Dora** or **Theodora.**

Doria *Gk.* Place name: "from Doris," an area in Greece. Also
   feminine of **Dorian;** variant of **Dorothy, Theodora** (*Gk.*
   "Gift from God").
   Dori, Dorian, Doriane, Dorria

Dorinda *Gk./Sp.* Variant of **Dora.** English poets in the 18th
   century coined a number of names with the "-inda" suffix.
   This is one of the more common.
   Derinda, Dorrinda

Doris (*Fem. Dorian*) *Gk.* Place name: "from Doris," an area
   in Greece. This form is more common than **Doria,** having
   been hugely popular between 1900 and the 1930s.
   Dori, Doria, Dorice, Dorisa, Dorrys

Dorothy *Gk.* "Gift of God." **Theodora,** never as popular,
   simply reverses the order of the Greek words. Has had two
   periods of popularity: around 1500 to 1700 and 1900 to
   the mid-1920s. The latter vogue may have been inspired

by the heroine of Frank Baum's *The Wonderful Wizard of Oz,* published in 1900.

> Dasha, Dasya, Dodie, Dody, Doe, Doll, Dollie, Dolly, Dora, Doretta, Dori, Dorit, Doro, Dorothea, Dorothée, Dorrit, Dorthea, Dorthy, Dot, Tea, Thea

Drusilla *Lat.* Feminine version of a Roman clan name that appears in the New Testament. Very unusual nowadays.

> Dru, Drucella, Drucilla, Druesilla

Duane *Ir. Gael.* "Swarthy." Dates from the 1940s. More common for boys.

> Duana, Duna, Dwana, Dwayna, Dwayne

Dulcie *Lat.* "Sweet." Roman name revived for some years at the turn of the 20th century but extremely unusual now. Cervantes used a slightly different form when he named the *Don Quixote* heroine **Dulcinea.**

> Delcina, Dulce, Dulcea, Dulcia, Dulciana, Dulcibella, Dulcine, Dulcinea, Dulcy

Dusty (*Fem.* **Dustin**) An English place name transferred to first name. Probably popularized in the 20th century by English singer Dusty Springfield.

> Dustee, Dustie, Dustin

Dylana (*Fem.* **Dylan**) *Welsh.* "Born from waves." Use of Dylan tends to be a tribute to the poet Dylan Thomas. Most parents today would not hesitate to use the original masculine name for a girl.

> Dillan, Dillon, Dylane, Dyllan

E

Ebony Name of the wood, which is prized for its black color. In use since the 1970s with African-American families.

> **Ebboney, Eboney, Eboni**

Echo *Gk.* Name of a mythological nymph who was a disembodied voice. One version of her story holds that she pined away for Narcissus until only her voice was left.

Eda *OE.* "Wealthy, happy." Also possibly a variation of **Edith.**

> **Ede**

Edana (*Fem.* **Aidan**) *Gael.* "Fire." Although Aidan is still primarily a boy's name (and chugging up the popularity charts at a rapid rate), it is increasingly used for girls as well.

> **Aidana, Aydana**

Eden *Heb.* "Pleasure, delight." It is a short step from the Hebrew meaning of the word to its general association with Paradise. The name is used infrequently for boys as well as girls.

> **Eaden, Eadin**

Edina *OE.* Possibly a form of **Edwina,** or a literary term meaning "from Edinburgh," the capital city of Scotland.

> **Adena, Adina**

Edith *OE.* "Prosperity/battle." Anglo-Saxon name that continued to be used after the Norman Conquest and was revived along with other ancient names in the 19th century. By the 1870s, it was one of the 10 most popular girls' names in Britain but has been steadily displaced since the 1930s.

> Dita, Eadie, Eadith, Ede, Edie, Edita, Editha, Edithe, Edyth, Eydie

Edna *Heb.* "Pleasure, enjoyment." Perhaps arising from the same root as **Eden.** First used in the 18th century but very popular in the last half of the 19th century, especially in the United States.

Edwina (*Fem.* **Edwin**) *OE.* "Wealth/friend." Feminine variant of an Anglo-Saxon name revived in the 19th century but never hugely popular.

> Edina, Edwinna, Edwyna

Effie *Gk.* "Pleasant speech." Short version of **Euphemia,** used as an independent name starting in the 1860s.

Eileen *Ir.* "Shining, brilliant." Form of **Helen.** Irish names were fashionable in England around 1870. By the 1920s, Eileen was one of the most popular girls' names in Britain.

> Aileen, Ailene, Aline, Ayleen, Eilleen, Ileene, Ilene

Ekaterina *Slavic.* Variation of **Catherine** (*Gk.* "Pure").

> Yekaterina

Elaine *OF.* "Bright, shining, light." Form of **Helen.** In the King Arthur myths, Elaine is a maiden who desperately loves

Lancelot. Tennyson's version of the tale has her dying
of this love, but in an earlier telling she actually has a
son—Galahad—by Lancelot.

> Alaina, Alayna, Alayne, Elaina, Elana, Elane,
> Elanna, Elayne, Ellayne, Lainey, Layney

Elberta (*Fem.* **Elbert**) *OE.* "Highborn/shining." Variant of
Alberta.

> Elbertha, Elberthe

Eleanor Possibly a form of **Helen** (*Gk.* "Light") or from a different Greek root meaning "clemency, mercy." The queen
of Henry II of England, Eleanor of Aquitaine, introduced the
name to England in the 13th century, and it has been used
steadily since, especially in the United States, under the
influence of much-loved First Lady Eleanor Roosevelt.

> Aleanor, Alenor, Allinor, Eileen, Elaine, Eleanora,
> Eleanore, Elen, Elena, Elenor, Elenora, Elenore,
> Eleonora, Eleonore, Elienora, Elinor, Elinore, Ella,
> Elleanora, Elle, Ellen, Ellene, Ellenore, Ellinor,
> Helenora, Leanora, Lenora, Lenore, Leonora,
> Leonore, Nell, Nellie, Nelly, Nora, Norah

Electra *Gk.* "Shining, bright." Though the name is derived
from the same roots as the word *electricity*, many people
will associate it with the Greek tragedies of the house of
Atreus told by Aeschylus, Euripides, Sophocles, and Eugene
O'Neill. All versions involve incest, murder, and vengeance.

Alectra, Elektra, Elettra, Ellektra

Elfrida *OE.* "Elf/power." Uncommon name. *See also* **Alfreda.**

Alfrida, Elfre, Elfredah, Elfredda, Elfrieda, Elfryda, Elva, Freeda, Frieda

Elga *Slavic.* "Sacred." *See also* **Olga.**

Elgiva, Ellga, Helga

Eliane (*Fem.* **Elias**) *Fr.* from *Heb.* "Jehovah is God."

Elia, Eliana, Elianna

Elidi *Gk.* "Gift of the sun."

Eliora *Heb.* "The Lord is my light."

Eleora, Eliorah, Elleora, Elliora

Elise *Fr.* Variation of **Elizabeth** (*Heb.* "Pledged to God").

Eliese, Elisa, Elize, Elyce, Elyse, Liese, Liesl, Lise

Elisheva *Heb.* "The Lord is my pledge."

Eliseva, Elisheba

Elissa Form of **Alice** or **Elizabeth.** First appeared around the 1930s.

Alissa, Alyssa, Elyssa, Elyssia, Ilyssa

Eliza Diminutive of **Elizabeth.** Frequently used in its own right from the 18th century onward. Especially popular in the first decade of the 20th century.

Aliza, Alizah, Elizah, Elyza, Liza

Elizabeth *Heb.* "Pledged to God." One of the 10 most popu-lar girls' names in the United States since 1980. Used in

full, it has a pleasant, old-fashioned ring, and it is a source
of endless diminutives and nicknames.

> Babette, Belle, Bess, Bessy, Beth, Betsey,
> Betsie, Bett, Betta, Bette, Bettina, Bettine, Betty,
> Bettye, Elisa, Elisabet, Elisabeth, Elisabetta,
> Elise, Elissa, Eliza, Elizabet, Elizabetta, Elle,
> Ellspet, Ellyse, Else, Elsie, Elspeth, Elyse,
> Elyssa, Elyza, Helsa, Ilsa, Isabel, Isobel, Leeza,
> Lib, Libbie, Libby, Lilibet, Lisa, Lisabeth, Lisbet,
> Lisbeth, Lise, Lisette, Lissa, Liz, Liza, Lizabeth,
> Lizette, Lizzy, Lysbeth, Ylisabet, Ysabel

Elke *Ger.* Variation of **Alice** (*OG.* "Noble, nobility"). Possibly
introduced to the English-speaking world by actress Elke
Sommer.

> Elka, Ellke, Ilka

Ella *OG.* "All, completely." Also possibly derived from **Alice,
Eleanor, Elizabeth.** Common in the Middle Ages and
revived in the United States in the late 19th century, but it
is now unusual.

> Ela, Ellie

Ellen Variant of **Helen** (*Gk.* "Shining, brightness"). Both forms
have been popular but rarely at the same time.

> Elen, Elena, Eleni, Elin, Ellene, Ellyn, Elyn

Elmira *Arab.* "Aristocratic lady." Also possibly a feminization of
Elmer (*OE.* "Highborn and renowned"). *See also* **Almira.**

> Almira, Ellmeria, Mera, Mira

Eloise *Fr.* form of **Louise** (*OG.* "Renowned in battle"). Made
   famous by the medieval love letters between Heloise and
   Abelard. Modern parents, though, are more likely to think
   of the madcap six-year-old denizen of New York's Plaza
   Hotel who stars in Kay Thompson's books for children.
   Aloysia, Eloisa, Heloise

Elsie Variant of **Elizabeth** via its Scottish form, **Elspeth**.
   Independently used since the 18th century and extremely
   popular in the United States by the late 19th century.
   Elsa, Elsee, Elsey, Elspeth

Elvira *Sp.* Meaning unclear, possibly a place name. Mostly
   literary use.
   Ellvira, Elva, Elvera

Emeline *OG.* Possibly "industrious." Possibly also a variant of
   Emily or **Amelia.**
   Emaline, Emelyn, Emiline

Emerald Jewel name. *See also* **Esmeralda.**

Emily *Lat.* Clan name. In spite of the similarity of form, it
   has a different root from **Amelia.** Naturally, many of the
   variants are very close. A hugely popular name in the 19th
   century, it lost status after 1900. But it has been the number one girls' name in the United States since 1996.
   **Amalia, Ameline, Em, Emalee, Emelia, Emelina,
   Emelyn, Emilia, Emlyn, Emmaline, Emmi, Milka**

Emma *OG.* "Embracing everything." Royal name in medieval
   England and hugely popular at the end of the 19th century.

Recently very fashionable in the United States, probably on the coattails of the evergreen **Emily**.

> Emelina, Emme, Emmie

Emmanuelle (*Fem.* **Emmanuel**) *Heb.* "God is among us."

> Emanuela, Emanuelle

Ena Short for names such as **Georgina** and **Regina**.

Enid *Welsh.* "Life, spirit." Name from the King Arthur myths revived mildly in the early 19th century and quite popular in England by the 1920s.

> Enyd

Erica (*Fem.* **Eric**) *Scan.* "Ruler forever." Though a staple in Scandinavia, it wasn't used in the English-speaking world until the late 19th century.

> Aerica, Ericka, Erika, Erykah, Eyrica, Ricki, Rikky

Erin *Ir. Gael.* "From the island to the west." Erin is a literary term for Ireland, hence the name's popularity among Irish-descended families. Ironically, it is not much used in Ireland itself.

> Aeran, Aerin, Airin, Eire, Eirin, Eryn

Erma Variant of **Irma** (*OG.* "Universal, complete"). Enjoyed a brief period of use from around 1890 to 1940.

> Irma

Ernestine (*Fem.* **Ernest**) *OE.* "Sincere." Use at the end of the 19th century follows the enormous popularity of **Ernest** for boys at that period.

> Erna, Ernesta, Ernestina

Esmée *Fr.* "Esteemed." Originally a male name brought to
  Scotland by a French cousin of James VI. Now used more
  for girls, though scarce.
  > Esmay, Esmé, Ismé

Esmeralda *Sp.* "Emerald." Jewel name first used in the
  1880s and more common than **Emerald.**
  > Emerald, Emeralda, Emeraldina, Emeraude,
  > Esmarelda, Esmeralda, Esmiralda

Esperanza *Sp.* "Hope."
  > Esperance, Esperantia

Estelle *OF.* "Star." French form of a name apparently coined
  by Charles Dickens for a character in his 1861 novel *Great
  Expectations. See also* **Astra; Esther; Stella.**
  > Essie, Estel, Estele, Estell, Estella, Estrella,
  > Estrellita, Stella

Esther *Per.* "Star." More particularly, the planet Venus. Esther
  in the Bible was an orphan named Hadassah who became
  the wife of King Ahasuerus under her new name.
  > Essie, Esta, Estée, Ester, Ettie, Hester, Hesther,
  > Hetty, Hittie

Ethel *OE.* "Noble." A short form of various old-fashioned
  names such as **Etheldreda.** First appeared on its own in
  the 1840s, and the name was very popular by the 1870s.
  Unlikely to be revived in the 21st century.
  > Ethelda, Ethelin, Ethelinda, Etheline, Ethlyn,
  > Ethyll

Etta Feminine diminutive suffix (**Georgette, Henriette**) that
has attained the status of an independent name.
Ettie, Etty

Eugenia (*Fem*. **Eugene**) *Gk*. "Wellborn." The French form,
Eugenie, was made famous by Napoleon III's beautiful
empress and has persisted in the European royal houses.
Eugenie, Evgenia, Geena, Gena, Genia

Eunice *Gk*. "Victorious." Biblical name: In the New Testament,
Eunice is the mother of Timothy.

Euphemia *Gk*. "Favorable speech." Early Christian name
borne by a 4th-century virgin martyr. The name was more
common in its short forms such as **Effie** through the 19th
century.
Effie, Effy, Eufemia, Euphemie

Evangeline *Gk*. "Good news." Derived from *evangel,* the
term that came to be used for the Gospels, or the four
New Testament accounts of Christ's life. First used in
English by Alfred Tennyson in his 1847 poem "Evangeline."
Eva, Evangelia, Evangelina, Evangelista

Eve *Heb*. "Life." In the form **Eva,** somewhat popular from
the mid-19th century, usually as a shortened version of
Evangeline. Eve, the French form of the name, is used
steadily but not in great numbers. A clever name for the
first girl in a family of boys.
Eva, Evaleen, Eveline, Evette, Evie, Evita

Evelina *OG.* or *OF.,* possibly "hazelnut." Norman import to
　　Britain, where it was brought to prominence by Fanny
　　Burney's popular novel *Evelina* in the 18th century.
　　Gradually overwhelmed by **Evelyn.**
　　　　Eveleen, Eveline, Evelyne
Evelyn *OG.* Obscure meaning, from the same root as
　　Evelina. Not, as it would seem, a combination of **Eve** and
　　Lynn, but originally a surname and later a boy's name.
　　　　Evaleen, Evalyn, Evelene, Eveline, Evelyne,
　　　　Evelynn, Evelynne
Evette *Fr.* Variant form of **Yvette,** in turn a diminutive of
　　Yvonne. Also used as a diminutive for **Eve,** though the
　　roots are different.
　　　　Eevette, Evetta, Eyvetta, Eyvette

Faith *ME.* "Loyalty." One of the most common of the virtue
　　names, along with **Hope** and **Charity.**
　　　　Fae, Faithe, Fay, Faye, Fé
Fallon *Ir. Gael.* "Descended from a ruler." Surname brought
　　to public notice and some popularity by a character on the
　　TV serial *Dynasty.*
　　　　Fallan, Fallen

Fanny (Diminutive of **Frances**) *Lat.* "From France." This form became extremely popular in the early 19th century and remained a favorite until around 1910, when its inexplicable adoption as a term for the buttocks extinguished it as a first name.

Fan, Fanney, Fannie

Fatima *Arab.* Meaning unclear, though Fatima was Mohammed's favorite daughter. According to the Koran, she was one of only four perfect women in the world.

Fateema, Fatimah, Fatma

Fawn *OF.* "Young deer." Names for girls have been drawn from various segments of the natural world—flowers, gems, seasons, months—but animal names, for some reason, are rarer.

Faun, Fawna

Fay *OF.* "Fairy." Or diminutive of **Faith.** First used in significant numbers in the 1920s.

Faye, Fée

Felicia (*Fem.* **Felix**) *Lat.* "Lucky, fortunate, happy." Thanks to the popular 1990s television series, **Felicity** is the most common form of this name.

Falicia, Falisha, Felice, Feliciana, Felicidad, Felicie, Felicienne, Félicité, Felicity, Felis, Felisa, Felisha, Feliss, Felita, Feliz, Feliza, Filicia, Phylicia, Phyllisha

Fernanda (*Fem.* **Ferdinand**) *OG.* Possibly "peace/courage" or "voyage/courage." Very rare feminine form of an equally rare male name.

> Anda, Annda, Ferdinanda, Ferdinande, Nan, Nanda

Filia *Gk.* "Friendship."

> Philia

Filippa Variation of **Philippa** (*Gk.* "Lover of horses").

Fiona *Ir. Gael.* "Fair, pale." Apparently coined by an English author at the turn of the 20th century, and its popularity in Britain has been growing since the 1930s.

> Ffion, Ffiona, Ffyona, Fione, Fionna, Fyona

Fionnula *Ir. Gael.* "White shoulder."

> Fenella, Finola, Fionnuala, Nola, Nuala

Flana *Ir. Gael.* "Russet hair."

> Flanagh, Flann, Flanna, Flannery

Flavia *Lat.* "Yellow hair." Originally a Latin clan name.

Fleur *Fr.* "Flower." In John Galsworthy's *The Forsyte Saga,* one of the principal characters is Fleur, which brought the name to some prominence. The BBC TV adaptation in the 1970s also provoked a spate of use.

> Fleurette, Fleurine

Flora *Lat.* "Flower." The name of the Roman goddess of springtime and of a 9th-century martyred saint. Flora Macdonald was a Scottish heroine who helped Bonnie

Prince Charlie escape the English. The name was naturally popular in Scotland and throughout England in the last half of the 19th century.

Fiorella, Floralia, Flore, Florida, Florie, Florine, Floris

Florence *Lat.* "In bloom." Used for both men and women until the 17th century, when it faded from sight. Modern use is almost entirely inspired by the fame of Florence Nightingale, who was actually named for the Italian city where she was born.

Fiorentina, Fiorenza, Flo, Flor, Flora, Florance, Flore, Florencia, Florencita, Florentia, Florentina, Florentyna, Florenza, Florenzia, Flori, Floria, Floriana, Florinda, Florine, Floris, Florrance, Florrie, Florry, Flossie, Flossy

Flower *OF.* "Blossom."

Frances (*Fem.* **Francis**) *Lat.* "From France." Until the 17th century, **Francis** was used for both sexes. Spelled with an "e," it was a very popular choice in the first quarter of the 20th century.

Fan, Fannie, Fanny, Fran, Francee, Franceline, Francesca, Francess, Francetta, Francey, Franchesca, Francie, Francine, Francisca, Franciska, Françoise, Franka, Frankie, Franky, Frannie, Franny, Franziska

Freda *OG.* "Peaceful." Diminutive of **Alfreda, Frederica,** and **Winifred.** Most popular at the end of the 19th century, when **Fred** was fashionable for men.

> Freeda, Freida, Frida, Frieda

Frederica *OG.* "Peaceful ruler." Following the popularity of **Frederic,** substantially used in the late 19th century but now unusual.

> Federica, Freddi, Freddie, Fredericka, Frederique, Fredrika, Friederike, Rica, Rickie, Rikki

Freya *Scan.* "Highborn lady." The goddess of love in Norse mythology, corresponding perhaps to the Roman Venus. Friday is named for her.

> Fraya

Gabrielle (*Fem.* **Gabriel**) *Heb.* "Heroine of God." Used in English-speaking countries since the early 1900s, though the Italian form, **Gabriella,** has been popular since the 1950s. Gabriel is an archangel who appears in Christian, Jewish, and Muslim texts.

> Gabbe, Gabbi, Gabbie, Gabriel, Gabriela,

Gabriell, Gabriella, Gabrila, Gabryella, Gaby, Gavi, Gavra, Gavrila, Gavrilla

Gaea *Gk.* "The earth."

Gaia, Gaiea

Gail *Heb.* "My father rejoices." A diminutive of **Abigail** with an unusually strong life of its own, dating from around 1940, with special popularity in the 1950s.

Gael, Gahl, Gaila, Gaile, Gal, Gale, Gayla, Gayle

Galina *Rus.* Variant of **Helen** (*Gk.* "Shining brightly"). Currently very popular in Russia.

Galya *Heb.* "The Lord has redeemed."

Galia, Gallia, Gallya

Gemma *It.* "Precious stone." Curiously, did not come into fashion with other jewel names in the late 19th century but is slightly popular now.

Jemma

Genevieve A name whose origin is unclear, but sources suggest possibly *OG.* "White wave"; *Celt.* "Race of women." Saint Genevieve, the patroness of Paris, was a 5th-century virgin who defended Paris against Attila the Hun, among others. Use in English-speaking countries has tended to simmer along at a low level.

Gena, Geneva, Genivieve, Genny, Genovera, Genoveva, Jenevieve, Jennie, Jenny

Georgia (*Fem.* George) *Lat.* "Farmer." The preferred feminine of George in the United States.

> Georgeanne, Georgeina, Georgena, Georgette,
> Georgiana, Georgianna, Georgianne, Georgina,
> Giorgia, Giorgyna, Jorgina, Jorja

Geraldine (*Fem.* **Gerald**) *OG./Fr.* "Spear ruler." Though the
form was coined in the 16th century, its real popularity
followed the fashion for Gerald in the mid-19th century
through the 1950s.

> Dina, Geralda, Geraldina, Geralyn, Geri, Gerri,
> Gerrilyn, Gerroldine, Gerry, Jeraldeen, Jere, Jeri,
> Jerilene

Gertrude *OG.* "Strength of a spear." An old name (there was
a 7th-century Saint Gertrude) revived to immense popularity with the late 19th-century fashion for the antique. Now
resoundingly out of style.

> Gerda, Gerta, Gertie, Gertrud, Gertruda, Gerty,
> Trude, Trudy

Ghaliya *Arab.* "Sweet smelling."

Gillian *Lat.* "Youthful." Anglicization of **Juliana.** A standard
name in the Middle Ages in England. Never widespread in
the United States, though its diminutive, **Jill,** had quite a
fashionable spell.

> Ghilian, Ghillian, Gilian, Giliana, Gill, Gillan,
> Gillie, Jillian, Jillianne, Jillyan

Gina Diminutive of **Regina** and **Angelina.** Also could be
considered a feminization of **Gene** or a variant of **Jean.**

Independent use dates from the 1920s, concentrated in the 1950s.

Geena, Gena, Ginette, Ginna, Jena, Jeena

Ginger *Lat.* "Ginger." Also can be a diminutive of **Virginia** (*Lat.* "Virgin"). Depends almost completely on the fame of actress Ginger Rogers, whose given name was Virginia.

Ginny Diminutive of **Virginia** (*Lat.* "Virgin").

Ginnie, Jinny

Giselle *OG.* "Pledge/hostage." Use may reflect a fondness for the famous 19th-century ballet whose tragic heroine is a peasant girl betrayed by a noble suitor.

Ghisele, Ghisella, Gisela, Gisele, Gisella

Gladys *Welsh.* Variant of **Claudia** (*Lat.* "Lame"). Suddenly glamorous in the late 19th century and used in several Edwardian romantic novels, which further heightened its appeal. Now rare.

Gladdys, Gwladys

Gloria *Lat.* "Glory." Apparently coined in 1898 by playwright George Bernard Shaw's *You Never Can Tell*. The exposure given to the name by actress Gloria Swanson was probably crucial to its popularity from the 1920s through the 1960s.

Glorea, Gloriana, Gloriane, Glorie

Grace *Lat.* "Grace." Originally had nothing to do with physical grace but rather with divine favor and mercy. Used in that sense by the Puritans and brought to the United States, where it was very fashionable at the end of the 19th century. Now one of the top 20 names in the United States, and the only one that's monosyllabic.

> Engracia, Gracey, Gracia, Graciana, Graciela, Gracina, Gratia, Gratiana, Grazia, Grazyna

Greta *Ger.* Diminutive of **Margaret** (*Gk.* "Pearl"). Most used during the 1930s, clearly inspired by Greta Garbo.

> Greeta, Gretchen, Gretel, Gretha, Grethel, Gretna, Gretta

Gretchen *Ger.* Diminutive of **Margaret** (*Gk.* "Pearl"). Used on its own in English-speaking countries in the 20th century.

Griselda *OG.* "Gray fighting maid." In a famous tale told by both Boccaccio and Chaucer, "Patient Griselda" is a meek wife who submits to numerous trials devised by her husband to test her submissiveness. The name has long since been eclipsed by its short form, **Zelda**.

> Grisel, Griseldis, Grizel, Grizelda, Gryselde, Gryzelde, Selda, Zelda

Guinevere *Welsh.* "White and smooth, soft." The name of King Arthur's ill-fated queen. The most common form today is **Jennifer**.

> Gaynor, Genever, Genevieve, Genevra, Geniffer, Genna, Gennifer, Genny, Ginevra, Guenever, Guenevere, Guinever, Gwen, Gweniver, Gwennie, Gwenore, Gwyn, Gwynn, Jen, Jeni, Jenifer, Jennie, Jennifer, Wendy, Winne, Winnie

Gwendolyn *Welsh.* "Fair bow." In some legends, Merlin the magician has a wife named Gwendolyn. The old Welsh name was revived in the late 19th century and is now rare, though its diminutive, **Wendy,** lingers on.

> Guendolen, Guendolynn, Gwen, Gwenda, Gwendaline, Gwendolen, Gwendolene, Gwendolin, Gwendolynne, Gwenna, Gwenette, Gwennie, Gwenyth, Gwyn, Wendie, Wynne

Gwyneth *Welsh.* "Happiness." Most popular in Wales and Britain in the 1930s and 1940s but never a strong name in the United States.

> Gweneth, Gwenyth, Gwineth, Gwynne, Gwynneth

Gwynn *Welsh.* "Fair, blessed." Also diminutive of **Gwendolyn** or **Gwyneth.**

> Gwin, Gwinna, Gwynne

Gypsy *OE.* The tribe of Romany was originally called gypsy because it was thought that it had originated in Egypt. Use of the name, as in the case of Gypsy Rose Lee, is more often as a nickname.

> Gipsee, Gipsy

Habibah *Arab.* "Loved one."
    Habiba, Habibi, Haviva
Hadria *Lat.* Place name: "From Adria." Variation of **Adrian.**
    Hadriana, Hadriane, Hadrienne
Hagar *Heb.* "Forsaken." In the Old Testament, Hagar is the
    handmaid of Abraham's barren wife, Sarah, and Sarah
    sends her away when she has a son by Abraham.
    Haggar, Hagir
Haidée *Gk.* "Modest." The name was brought to public
    knowledge by Byron, who used it in his poem "Don Juan."
Hailey *OE.* "Hay meadow." This name and **Hallie,** in their
    various spellings, have become very popular recently.
    Haley and Hailey are entered as different names on the
    Social Security Administration's list of popular names, but
    combined, they would probably number just below the
    top 10.
    Halea, Haleigh, Hailey, Hayley
Halimah *Arab.* "Gentle, soft spoken."
    Haleema, Halima
Halimeda *Gk.* "Thinking of the sea."
    Halameda, Halette, Hali, Hallie, Meda, Medie
Hallie (*Fem.* **Henry**) *OG.* "Ruler of the home or estate." Hallie

is considered a form of **Harriet,** as **Hal** is a nickname for
Harry. Parents probably don't differentiate, though, between Hallie and the very similar and fashionable **Hailey.**

    Hali, Halle, Hallee, Halley

Hana *Jap.* "Flower."

    Hanae, Hanako

Hannah *Heb.* "Grace." In the Old Testament, Hannah is the
mother of the prophet Samuel. The name was steadily
popular from around 1600 through the 19th century,
peaking around 1800. Hannah has been a top 10 favorite
in the United States since the mid-nineties, eclipsing all
European forms of the name except **Anna.**

    Ann, Anna, Anne, Annie, Chana, Chanah,
    Channach, Hana, Hanna, Hanne, Hannele,
    Hannelore, Hannie, Hanny, Nan, Nanny

Happy *Eng.* "Cheerful, lighthearted." Though it was common
enough in the 19th century, **Felicity, Hilary, Joy** or even
Bliss are now more likely to be used now. Happy does
occur as a nickname.

Harley *OE.* Place name: "The long field." Familiar to most
people as half of the name of a great motorcycle, the
Harley-Davidson. Fairly frequent use as a girl's name is
probably influenced by its fashionable sound.

    Arlea, Arlee, Arleigh, Arley, Harlea, Harlee,
    Harleigh, Harlie, Harly

Harmony *Lat.* "Harmony."

> **Harmonia, Harmonie**

Harriet *(Fem. Henry) OG.* "Ruler of the home or estate." An informal version of **Henrietta,** very popular in the 18th and 19th centuries, and after nearly a century of obscurity, ready for a revival.

> **Hallie, Harrie, Harriett, Harrietta, Harriette, Harriot, Harriott, Hatsey, Hatsie, Hatsy, Hatty**

Hayley *OE.* Place name: "hay meadow." Other sources suggest derivation from a Norse word, *haela,* which means "hero." Probably neither meaning nor history contributes much to the recent popularity of this name, which was made famous by actress Hayley Mills in the 1960s. Both **Hailey** and **Haley** are more fashionable spellings.

> **Haeley, Hailea, Hailee, Haileigh, Haleigh, Halie, Hally, Haylea, Hayleigh**

Hazel *OE.* Tree name. The late 19th-century vogue for botanical names tended to concentrate on flowers rather than trees; Hazel is an exception.

> **Hazelle, Hazle**

Heather *ME.* Flower name. Introduced with other botanical names in the late 19th century but really took off in the late 20th century. A top 10 name in the 1970s, which means that many of today's mothers are named Heather.

Hedda *OG.* "Warfare." The more common anglicized version
of **Hedwig**.

> Heda, Heddie, Hedi, Hedvige, Hedwig, Hedwiga,
> Hedy, Hetta

Heidi Diminutive of **Adelaide** (*OG.* "Noble, nobility"). Made
popular by Johanna Spyri's famous novel of 1881, first
in German-speaking countries, later in the United States.
Its surge of popularity in the 1970s may have been influenced by a highly publicized TV production of the late
1960s.

> Heida, Heide

Helen *Gk.* "Light." The most famous Helen is probably Helen
of Troy, the daughter of Zeus by Leda. In some story versions, her phenomenal beauty was the root cause of the
Trojan War; hers was "the face that launched a thousand
ships." The name has been understandably popular
through the ages and has spawned many variants, of which
Eleanor is the most common.

> Aileen, Ailene, Aleanor, Aline, Eileen, Elaina,
> Elaine, Elana, Elayne, Eleanor, Eleanore, Elena,
> Eleni, Elenora, Eleonora, Elianora, Elinor, Ella,
> Elle, Ellen, Ellenora, Ellie, Ellinor, Ellyn, Galina,
> Helena, Hélène, Helenore, Helia, Hella, Hellene,
> Hellia, Ileana, Ilene, Jelena, Lana, Leanora,
> Lena, Lenore, Leonora, Leonore, Lina, Nell,
> Nelly, Nonnie, Nora, Yelena

Helga *OG.* "Holy, sacred." Variation of **Olga**.

    Helge, Hellga, Hellge

Heloise *Fr.* Variant of **Louise** (*OG.* "Renowned in war"). The 12th-century French philosopher Pierre Abelard fell in love with and seduced his student Heloise. Her uncle and guardian had him emasculated, even though he married Heloise. She became a nun, he a monk.

    Aloysia, Eloisa, Eloise, Lois

Henrietta (*Fem.* **Henry**) *OG.* "Ruler of the house." More formal version of **Harriet** that briefly became popular at the turn of the 20th century.

    Enriqueta, Etta, Etty, Hattie, Hendrika, Henriette, Hettie

Hermione *Gk.* "Earthly."

    Hermia, Hermina

Hester *Gk.* "Star." Variation of **Esther**. The most famous Hester is probably the adulteress in Hawthorne's *The Scarlet Letter,* Hester Prynne.

    Hesther, Hestia, Hetty

Hilda *OG.* "Battle woman." One of the Valkyrie of Teutonic legend was named Hilda. A medieval name with a Victorian revival that lasted through the 1930s. Now unusual.

    Hilde, Hildie, Hildy

Hillary *Gk.* "Cheerful, happy." The name comes from the same root as the word *hilarious.* The name was used for boys until the 17th century, but the late 19th-century re-

vival made it generally a girl's name, which was especially
fashionable in the 1950s.

    Hilaria, Hilarie, Hilary

Holly *OE.* Botanical name. First used at the turn of the 20th
century and newly popular in the 1960s. Obviously a sea-
sonal favorite most intensively used in December.

    Holley, Hollie

Honey *OE.* The word, or endearment, used as a name.

Honora *Lat.* "Woman of honor." As **Honour,** used by the
Puritans (along with other abstract concepts such as
Constance). **Honoria** was more common in the 18th
century.

    Honor, Honoria, Honour

Hope *OE.* "Hope." One of the three cardinal virtues, along with
Faith and **Charity.**

Hyacinth *Gk.* Flower name. There was a 3rd-century saint
of this name, which was used for boys as well as girls. In
Greek legend, Apollo loved a beautiful youth of this name;
the hyacinth flower sprang up from his blood when he
died.

    Cintha, Cinthia, Giacinta, Hyacintha, Hyacinthe,
    Jacinta

Ida Meaning unclear: possibly *OE.* "Prosperous, happy"; *OG.* "Hardworking." Very fashionable at the turn of the 20th century in the United States.
   Idah, Idalene, Idalina
Ieesha Variation of **Aisha** (*Arab.* "Woman"; *Swahili.* "Life").
   Eyeesha, Ieasha, Ieashia
Ilana *Heb.* "Tree."
   Elana, Elanit, Ileana
Ilene Modern variant of **Aileen** (*Gk.* "Light").
   Ileen, Illeene
Iliana *Gk.* "Trojan." The poetic name for the ancient city of Troy was Ilion.
   Ileana, Ileanna, Illeanna, Illia
Imelda *OG./It.* "All-consuming fight." A name occasionally used (especially in Catholic families, after a virgin saint) until the explosive fame of Philippine First Lady Imelda Marcos. Now it seems slated for a long period of neglect.
   Amelda, Imalda, Ymelda
Immaculada *Sp.* "Without stain." A reference to the Immaculate Conception.
   Imaculada, Immaculata
Imogen *Lat.* Some sources claim it means "last born,"

whereas others suggest "image," while still another traces it back to "innocent." Despite Shakespeare's use of the name, it was obscure until the 20th century.

Imogene, Imogenia

Ina *Lat.* Suffix to make male names feminine, as in **Clementina** or **Edwina**. Used independently since the Victorian era.

Ena, Yna

India Country name. Like any pretty geographic name, could be used by parents who have a special attachment to the country.

Indya

Inez *Sp.* Variant of **Agnes** (*Lat.* "Pure"). Unusual in English-speaking countries.

Ines, Inesita, Inessa, Ynes

Inga *Scan.* "Guarded by Ing." In Norse mythology, Ing was a powerful god of fertility and peace. His name is an element in several modern names such as **Ingrid** and **Ingmar.**

Inge, Ingeborg

Ingrid *Scan.* "Beautiful." The most popular of the "Ing" names, doubtless because of the fame of Swedish actress Ingrid Bergman.

Inga, Inge, Inger, Ingmar

Inocencia *Sp.* "Innocence."

Innocencia, Inocenta

Iolanthe *Gk.* "Violet flower." The more common form is the Spanish variant, **Yolanda.** Gilbert and Sullivan's 1882 operetta *Iolanthe* did little to popularize this form.

Iolanda, Iolanta, Iolantha, Jolantha, Jolanthe

Iona *Gk.* Place name. Island off the coast of Scotland, site of an early monastery. Use as a name is mostly Scottish.

Ione *Gk.* "Violet." Flower name in an exotic form.

Ionia, Ionie

Irene *Gk.* "Peace." Very common under the Roman Empire, but it first appeared in English-speaking countries in the mid-19th century. It caught on quickly and was very popular in the first quarter of the 20th century.

Eirene, Ira, Irena, Irénée, Irina

Iris *Gk.* "Rainbow." Also (and this is probably the source of its popularity) name of a flower. Its use was established and faded with other flower names from around 1890 to the 1920s.

Irida, Iridiana

Irma *OG.* "Universal, complete." Rare now but used somewhat in the first part of the 20th century.

Erma, Irmina, Irmine

Isabella *Sp.* Variation of **Elizabeth** (*Heb.* "Pledged to God"). Most fashionable in the last quarter of the 19th century and once again in the top 10 in the United States. **Belle** and **Bella** are also independently used, probably because

of their own attractive meaning ("beautiful") in French and
Spanish.

**Bella, Belle, Isa, Isabeau, Isabel, Isabelita,
Isabell, Isabelle, Ishbel, Isobel, Isobell, Izzy,
Ysabel, Ysabella, Ysobel**

Isadora (*Fem.* **Isidore**) *Lat.* "Gift of Isis." Isis was the principal goddess of ancient Egypt, and Isidore was a popular
name among the ancient Greeks. The most famous Isadora
was, of course, modern dance pioneer Isadora Duncan.

Isidora, Ysadora

Isolde Meaning unclear, though some sources offer Welsh
for "fair lady." In legend Isolde is an Irish princess loved
by Tristan, but she marries his uncle, King Mark. The most
famous version of the tale is probably Wagner's opera
Tristan und Isolde.

Iseult, Iseut, Isolda, Isolt

Ivana (*Fem.* **Ivan**) Slavic Variation of **John** (*Heb.* "Jehovah is
gracious").

Iva, Ivanka, Ivanna

Ivy *OE.* Botanical name. Most popular in the first quarter of the
20th century.

Ivee, Ivey, Ivie

J

Jacinda *Sp.* Variation of **Hyacinth** (*Gk.* Flower name). There
was a 3rd-century Saint Hyacinth, and the name was used
for boys as well as girls. In Greek legend Apollo loved a
beautiful youth of the name; the hyacinth flower sprang up
from his blood when he died.

> Giacinda, Giacintha, Jacenta, Jacinta, Jacinthe

Jacqueline *Fr.* Diminutive of **Jacob** (*Heb.* "He who supplants"). Existed in Britain as early as the 17th century
but used in numbers only from the beginning of the 20th
century. In the United States, parents choosing it may
have been inspired by glamorous First Lady Jacqueline
Kennedy.

> Jacalyn, Jackelyn, Jacki, Jackie, Jaclin, Jaclyn,
> Jacquelean, Jacquelin, Jacquenetta, Jacquette,
> Jaqueline

Jade *Sp.* Jewel name, for the semiprecious green stone.
Perhaps because the jewel comes from the Orient, the
name has a vaguely exotic air.

> Jada, Jaida, Jayde

Jaffa *Heb.* "Beautiful." Also a place name: an ancient city that
served as the port for Tel Aviv.

> Jafit, Joppa

Jamie (*Fem.* **James**) *Heb.* "He who supplants." Also used as
a boy's name, but once a name becomes entrenched as
a feminine choice, parents tend to avoid it for their male
children.

> Jaime, Jaimee, Jaimey, Jamee, Jaymie

Jamila *Arab.* "Lovely."

> Jameela, Jameila

Jan (*Fem.* **John**) *Heb.* "The Lord is gracious."

> Jana, Janah, Janina, Janine, Jann, Janna

Jane (*Fem.* **John**) *Heb.* "The Lord is gracious." This is the
simplest current variant of **John** (though **Joan** predates
it), popular since the 16th century. It has been a tried-and-
true standby such as **Mary** or **Katherine,** as demonstrat-
ed by its number of variants. When many women at a time
shared the same name, variants sprang up to differentiate
them from one another; hence **Janelle, Janet, Janine,**
and so on.

> Gianina, Giovanna, Ivana, Jaine, Jan, Jana,
> Janeane, Janeen, Janella, Janelle, Janet,
> Janice, Janie, Janina, Janine, Janis, Janna,
> Jayne, Jean, Jeanette, Jeanie, Jeanne, Joana,
> Joanna, Johanna, Johnetta, Johnna, Joni,
> Juana, Juanita, Sheena

Janet The most common diminutive form of **Jane** is Janet,
but other forms such as **Janeta** and **Jonet** preceded it.

Janet was originally mostly Scottish, and was very popular in the 1950s.

> Gianetta, Janeta, Janetta, Jannet, Jenette

Janice Variant of **Jane.** Coined at the turn of the 20th century, in general circulation by the thirties and popular in the fifties.

> Janess, Janesse, Janiece, Janis, Jeniece

Jasmine *Per.* "Jasmine flower." Flower name with exotic connotations. The turn-of-the-20th-century vogue for flower names had its source in the English upper class. Jasmine became fashionable a bit later, in the 1930s, and has hovered just below top 20 use since 1990.

> Ismenia, Jasmin, Jasmina, Jassamayn, Jazmon, Jess, Jessamine, Jessamy, Jessamyn, Yasmeen, Yasmin, Yasmina, Yasmine

Jean Variation of **Jane.** Scottish origin, unusual elsewhere until the turn of the 20th century; most popular in the 1930s. Now preferred for boys, probably among United States Francophone populations, as it is a French version of **John.**

> Gene, Jeane, Jeanine, Jeanne, Jeannette, Jeannine, Jenette

Jelena *Rus.* Variant of **Helen** (*Gk.* "Light").

> Galina, Yelena

Jemima *Heb.* "Dove." Old Testament name: Jemima was one

of the three beautiful daughters of the persecuted Job. The
Puritans brought the name to the United States, where it is
now probably most familiar because of the Aunt Jemima
brand name for pancake mix and syrup.

> **Jemimah**

Jenna Diminutive of **Jennifer** or variant of **Jean** (*Heb.* "The
Lord is gracious"). Made famous by a character on *Dallas*,
played by Priscilla Presley. Quite well used.

> **Jena**

Jennifer *Welsh.* "White and smooth, soft." The modern and
most popular form of **Guinevere,** originally a Cornish
variant. The name held the number one spot in the United
States between 1970 and 1984.

> **Gennifer, Jen, Jenefer, Jeni, Jenifer, Jennie,**
> **Jenny**

Jerrie *OG./Fr.* "Spear ruler." Diminutive of **Geraldine.**

> **Jeree, Jeri**

Jessica *Heb.* "He sees." Coined by Shakespeare from the Old
Testament Iscah or Jesca. His Jessica was the daughter of
Shylock in *The Merchant of Venice*. Having been one of
the top three names in the United States since 1981, it is
now quickly losing favor.

> **Jess, Jessa, Jessaca, Jesse, Jessie, Jessika,**
> **Jessy**

Jewel *OF.* Word as first name. Though the vogue for jewel names occurred at the turn of the 20th century (along with the flower name fashion), Jewel came into use a little later, in the 1930s.

    Jewell

Jill Diminutive of **Gillian,** ultimately of **Juliana** (*Lat.* "Youthful"). Jill was popular before the 17th century and revived to widespread use after the 1920s.

    Jil, Jilian, Jilly

Joan (*Fem.* **John**) *Heb.* "The Lord is gracious." The medieval feminine version of John; Jeanne d'Arc's first name, for instance, was translated as Joan, the popular English equivalent of **Jeanne.** It was neglected for **Jane** by the 17th century. A brief intense revival occurred early in the 20th century for a score of years, but Joan is again widely neglected.

    Joane, Jonee, Joni

Joanna Variation of **Jane** or **Joan.** Its 19th-century use increased with the revival of Joan and continued to grow in the United States until around 1950. **Joanne,** the French form, was hugely popular in Britain in the 1970s.

    Joana, Jo Ann, Joanne, Johanna, Johnna, Jonna

Jocelyn Derivation unclear; possibly *OG.,* possibly *Lat.* "Cheerful." It was a man's name in the Middle Ages, revived as a girl's name in the early 20th century.

    Jocelin, Joceline, Joscelyn, Joss, Josslyn

Jody Diminutive of **Joan** and **Judith**. Used mostly since the
1950s in the United States.

> **Jodi, Jodie**

Joelle (*Fem.* **Joel**) *Heb.* "Jehovah is the Lord." Probably
popularized by a vogue for combined forms beginning with
"Jo-," such as **Joanne.** Reached its peak in the 1960s.

> **Joell, Joella, Joely**

Jordana *Heb.* "Descend." Named after the River Jordan. As a
boy's name, **Jordan** was first used in the Middle Ages by
Crusaders returning from the Holy Land.

> **Giordanna, Jordanna, Jordyn, Jourdan**

Josephine (*Fem.* **Joseph**) *Heb.* "Jehovah increases."
Napoleon's famous Empress Josephine's real name was
Marie Josephe (for the parents of Jesus), but Josephine
was used as a diminutive. It did not become fashionable
until the mid-19th century.

> **Fifi, Fifine, Guiseppina, Jo, Josanna, Josefa,
> Josefena, Josefina, Josette, Josey, Josiane,
> Josy**

Joy *Lat.* "Joy." Used in the Middle Ages and sparingly by
the Puritans, then revived at the turn of the 20th century.
Unusual after the height of its popularity in the 1950s.

> **Gioia, Gioya, Joie**

Joyce *Lat.* "Joyous." Used in the Middle Ages but nearly died
out until the early years of the 20th century, when it had a

spurt of immense popularity, especially in Britain.

> Joice, Joycelyn

Judith *Heb.* "Jewish." Old Testament name overlooked by the Puritans in their quest for girls' names but fashionable from the 1920s through the 1950s. In the Apocrypha, Judith is a Jewish heroine who decapitates the Assyrian general Holofernes and shows his head to the Hebrew army, inciting them to victory.

> Giuditta, Jodie, Judee, Judi, Judie, Judit, Judithe, Judy

Judy Diminutive of **Judith.** Dates back to the 18th century, but its true popularity follows that of Judith in the 20th century.

> Judee, Judi, Judie

Julia (*Fem. Julius*) *Lat.* Clan name. "Youthful." Along with **Juliana,** used among the early Christians, but it was rare in the Middle Ages. Since the 1700s, it has gone mildly in and out of fashion without ever being a tremendous favorite. In the 20th century, **Julie** was much more popular, but the European form with the "-a" ending has soared to frequent use since the mid-1990s. As **Juliet** the name is scarce.

> Giulia, Giuliana, Giulietta, Joletta, Julee, Juli, Juliana, Juliane, Julie, Julienne, Juliet, July, Julyanna, Yuliya

Juliana (*Fem.* **Julian**) *Lat.* Clan name. "Youthful." Appeared
in the early Christian era, and medieval use contracted it to
Gillian (and from there to **Jill**).

> **Giuliana, Juliane, Julianne, Julyana**

Julie *Fr.* Diminutive of **Julia** (*Lat.* Clan name. "Youthful").
Imported from France in the 1920s.

June Month used as name.

Juno *Lat.* "Queen of heaven." Juno was the Roman equivalent
of Hera in classical mythology: Jupiter's wife and the gods'
queen.

> **Juneau, Juneaux, Junot**

Justine *Lat.* "Fair, righteous." **Justina** was the original form,
but the French version took over in the 1960s.

> **Giustina, Justina**

Kaitlyn Variant of **Caitlin**, Irish form of **Katherine** (*Gk.*
"Pure"). A name as popular as Katherine has produced
endless variations over the years, and recently Caitlin and
its variants have become just as popular as the more
familiar form.

> **Caitlin, Caitlyn, Katelyn, Kathlin, Kathlyn**

Kalila *Arab.* "Beloved."

    Kalilah

Kalliope *Gk.* Calliope was the muse of epic poetry in Greek mythology.

Kallista *Gk.* "Most beautiful." Many of the "C" names that come from the Greek are spelled with a "K" in their original form.

    Callie, Callista, Kalista

Kamila *Arab.* "Perfect."

    Kamilah

Karen *Dan.* Variation of **Katherine** (*Gk.* "Pure"). Took hold in the 1930s in English-speaking countries and blossomed to great popularity in the 1950s and 1960s.

    Caren, Caron, Carynn, Karin, Keryn

Karima *Arab.* "Giving."

    Karimah

Karma *Hindi.* "Destiny, spiritual force." A New Age name if ever there was one.

Kate Diminutive of **Katherine.** Long-standing independent name, especially popular in the late 19th century.

    Cate, Catie, Kaethe, Katie, Katy

Katherine *Gk.* "Pure." One of the oldest recorded names, with roots in Greek antiquity. Almost every Western country has its own form of the name, and phonetic variations are endless. It has been borne by such illustrious women as Saint Catherine of Alexandria, the early martyr who was tortured on a spiked wheel; Empress Catherine the Great of Russia; and three of Henry VIII's six wives. The "K" spelling is much more popular in the United States than the "C" spelling. The variants here are a tiny sample of available forms of this name.

Caitlin, Caitriona, Caitrionagh, Cat, Catalin, Catalina, Catarina, Cate, Catharin, Catherine, Catheryn, Cathleen, Cathrynn, Cathy, Catrina, Ekaterina, Kaatje, Kaitlin, Katalin, Kate, Katelle, Katerina, Katha, Katharine, Katheryn, Kathie, Kathiryn, Kathleen, Kathlyne, Kathryn, Kathy, Kati, Katie, Katla, Katouska, Katrena, Katrien, Katrina, Katy, Katya, Kay, Kaye, Kit, Kittie, Kitty, Trina, Trinette, Yekaterina

Kathleen *Ir.* Variant of **Katherine** (*Gk.* "Pure"). Its use outside of Ireland began in the 1840s and may have been influenced by the great wave of Irish emigration sparked by the potato famines of those years.

Cathleen, Kaitlin, Katha, Kathaleen, Kathelina, Kathlin, Katlin

Katrina Variant of **Katherine** (*Gk.* "Pure"). Appealing for its European sound.

Caitrionagh, Catrina, Catriona, Katriona, Ketrina

Kay Diminutive of **Katherine**. First appeared at the turn of the 20th century but widespread in the middle of the century.

Caye, Kai, Kaye

Kayla Modern variant of **Katherine** (*Gk.* "Pure") or diminutive
of **Michaela** (*Heb.* "Who is like the Lord?"). After being
very fashionable in the 1980s, it is still steadily used, along
with a constellation of similar-sounding names (**Maya,
Lila, Kyla**).

  Cayla, Caylie, Kaela

Keisha Modern name, possibly formed as a short version of
Lakeisha, which in turn may be a variant of **Aisha** (*Arab.*
"Woman").

  Keasha, Keishah, Keshia

Kelly *Ir. Gael.* "Battle maid." Originally a very common Irish
last name and very popular as a girl's first name from
about the 1950s, peaking in the 1970s in the United
States.

  Kelley, Kelli

Kenya Place name used as first name.

  Kenia, Kennya

Kerry *Ir.* Place name: Kerry is a county in southwestern
Ireland. Also, according to some sources, *Ir. Gael.* "Dark-
haired."

  Keri, Kerrey, Kerrie

Kim Diminutive of **Kimberly.** Used as an independent name
from the mid-20th century, influenced by the careers of
actresses Kim Novak and Kim Basinger.

  Kimm, Kym

Kimberly *OE.* Place name. The "-y" suffix indicates a meadow. *The Facts on File Dictionary of First Names* traces the masculine use of the name to the Boer War, when many English soldiers were fighting in the South African town of Kimberley. It was used for girls after 1940 and became a great favorite in the 1960s and 1970s.

> Kimba, Kimber, Kimberlee, Kimberleigh, Kimberley, Kym, Kymberleigh

Kira Variation of **Kyra** (*Gk.* "Lady").

> Kiera

Kirsten *Scan.* Variant of **Christine** (*Gk.* "Christian"). Used generally from 1940, though the Scots had adopted this form long ago (possibly because of their geographical proximity to Scandinavia).

> Keirstin, Kierstin, Kirsti, Kirstie, Kirstin, Kirsty

Kitty Diminutive of **Katherine** (*Gk.* "Pure"). Used independently before the 16th century and during the 18th and 19th centuries. In the intervening two hundred years, it was a slang term for a woman of dubious morals.

> Kit, Kittee, Kittey

Kristen Combination of **Kirsten** and **Kristina**, variation of **Christine** (*Gk.* "Anointed, Christian.") Looks Scandinavian but isn't. Popular since the 1950s, along with similar forms such as **Kristin** and **Kristine**.

> Krissie, Krissy, Krista, Kristan, Kristeen,

Kristelle, Kristi, Kristina, Kristine, Kristyn, Kristyna, Krysta

Krystal Variant of **Crystal** (*Gk.* "Ice"). Transferred use of the word, mostly modern, and increasing since the 1950s. The "K" spelling is a recent variation, perhaps prompted by the *Dynasty* character Krystle Carrington.

Cristalle, Khrystle, Kristle, Krystal, Krystaline, Krystalle, Krystalline, Krystle

Kyla *Fem.* **Kyle** (*Scot.* Place name: "narrow spit of land"). Well-traveled parents may have crossed the Kyle of Lochalsh to reach the Isle of Skye.

Kyle

Kylie *Fem.* **Kyle.**

Kiley, Kylee, Kyley

Kyra *Gk.* "Lady." A contraction of *Kyria,* the Greek title of respect for a woman.

Kaira, Keera, Keira, Kira, Kyria

Lacey *OF.* Place name of obscure meaning, used as a boy's name in the 19th century and increasingly for girls today.

Lacee, Laci, Lacie, Laicey

Laila *Arab.* "Night." Usually taken to indicate dark hair or a dark complexion. *See also* **Leila**.

> Lailah, Layla, Laylah

Lainey Diminutive of **Elaine** (*OF.* "Bright, shining, light").

> Laney

Lakeisha Popular modern name made up of elements in vogue in the 1980s, the fashionable "La-" prefix attached to **Aisha** (*Arab.* "Woman").

> Lakecia, Lakeesha, Lekeesha

Lana Variant of **Helen** (*Gk.* "Light") or **Alanna** (*Gael.* "Rock" or "comely").

> Lanette, Lanna

Lani *Haw.* "Sky."

Lara Unclear origin. Some sources suggest *Lat.* "Famous"; others trace the name to the Greek **Larissa**.

> Larina, Larra

Larissa *Gk.* "Lighthearted." From the same root as **Hilary**.

> Larisa, Laryssa

Latanya Modern combined form: the "La-" prefix added to **Tanya**.

> Latania, Latonya

Latifah *Arab.* "Gentle, pleasant."

> Lateefa, Lateefah, Latifa

Laura *Lat.* "Laurel." In classical times, a crown made from the leaves of the bay, laurel was given to heroes or victors. The greatest popularity of the name came at the mid- to late

19th century, and it has remained quite a steady favorite ever since.

>Lauralee, Laure, Lauren, Laurena, Laurence, Laurentia, Laurentine, Lauretta, Lauri, Lauriane, Laurie, Laurina, Laurinda, Laurine, Lolly, Lora, Loree, Loreen, Loren, Lorene, Lorenza, Loretta, Lorette, Lori, Lorie, Lorinda, Lorri, Lorrie

Laurel *Lat.* "Laurel tree." Nature name whose popularity has coasted on the coattails of **Laura**, especially in the 20th century.

>Laural, Lauralle, Laurell

Lauren Variation of **Laura** or feminization of **Lawrence**. Introduced to the public by Lauren Bacall and immediately popular probably because the streamlined "modern" character of the name struck a chord in the 1940s. It has hovered in the 20 most popular American girls' names since 1990.

>Laren, Larren, Larrynn, Laryn, Lauryn, Loren, Lorin, Lorne, Lorren

Laverne *Lat.* Classical goddess of minor criminals, though the parents who made this name mildly popular in the 20th century probably didn't know that. It sounds enough like the romance languages' word for "green" (*vert, verde*) to have acquired misplaced connotations of green trees or springtime.

>Lavern, Laverna

Lavinia *Lat.* "Woman of Rome." Classical name.

> Lavina, Lavinie, Livinia

Leah *Heb.* "Weary." Old Testament name: Leah was the wife of Jacob, married to him by a ruse in the place of her sister, Rachel. Used with considerable steadiness.

> Lea, Liyah

Lee *OE.* Place name: "pasture or meadow." One of the few truly unisex names. The tenacious masculine hold on Lee may have been helped by tough-guy actor Lee Marvin.

> Lea, Leigh

Leila *Arab.* "Night." Used by authors in the early 19th century for exotic female characters and more widely by American parents later in the century.

> Layla, Leela, Leilah, Leilia, Lela, Lelah, Leyla

Leilani *Haw.* "Flower from heaven."

Lena *Lat.* Diminutive of names such as **Helena**, **Caroline**, and **Marlene**.

> Lina

Lenore *Gk.* "Light." Variation of **Eleanor**.

> Lenor, Lenora, Leonora, Leonore

Leona (*Fem.* **Leon**) *Lat.* "Lion." American version; **Léonie** is more popular in Europe.

> Leone, Leonia, Léonie, Leontyne

Leslie *Scot. Gael.* Place name. Some sources suggest "the gray castle." Became a last name, then (in the 18th cen-

tury) a first name used for boys and girls. Boys' use has
been tied to admiration for actor Leslie Howard and is
more common in Britain.

Leslee, Lesley, Lesli, Lezlee

Letitia *Lat.* "Joy, gladness." In medieval England, the form
was **Lettice,** which survived into the 20th century.

Laetitia, Laetizia, Latisha, Leticia, Lettice, Lettie

Liana *Fr.* "To twine around." Can also be a diminutive of
Italianate names such as **Ceciliana** and **Silviana.**

Leana, Liane

Libby Diminutive of **Elizabeth** (*Heb.* "Pledged to God").

**Lib, Libbee, Libbey, Libbie, Libet, Liby, Lilibet,
Lilibeth**

Liberty *ME.* "Freedom."

Liese Diminutive of **Elizabeth** (*Heb.* "Pledged to God").
Mostly found in Germany.

Liesa, Lieselotte

Lila *Arab.* "Night." *See also* **Leila.**

Layla, Leila

Lillian *Lat.* "Lily." Very common variation of the flower name,
flourishing at the turn of the 19th and 20th centuries.

Lilia, Lilian, Liliane, Lilias, Lillyanne

Lily *Lat.* Flower name. Possibly because the lily plays such a
large part in Christian iconography, this has been one of
the most popular of the flower names and has produced

many variants. Ripe for a revival among parents with a
taste for nostalgia.

> Leelee, Lil, Lili, Lilia, Lilley, Lilli, Lillie, Lilly,
> Lilyan

Lina Diminutive of names ending with "-line" or "-lena," such
as **Caroline, Helena,** and **Marlene.** Variation of **Lena.**

> Leena, Leina

Linda *Sp.* "Pretty." Though the name existed as a particle of
other English names (**Belinda, Melinda**) by the time of its
great vogue in the 20th century (late 1930s to 1960s), it
was probably interpreted as "pretty." Rather neglected now.

> Lin, Lindey, Lindi, Lindie, Lindy, Lynda, Lynde,
> Lyndy, Lynnda, Lynndie

Lindsay *OE.* Place name: "island of linden trees." Originally a
surname used for boys until the middle of the 20th century but quite popular as a girl's name in the 1980s and
1990s. Use has tapered off.

> Lindsea, Lindsee, Lindsey, Lindsy, Linsay,
> Linsey, Linsie, Linzy, Linzee, Linzy, Lyndsay,
> Lyndsey, Lyndsie, Lynsey

Linette *Welsh.* "Idol"; *OF.* "Linnet" (a small bird). In historical terms, probably a variant of **Lynette,** which is not,
surprisingly enough, a form of **Lynn.** These names and
their variations were most popular from the 1940s into
the 1960s.

> Lenette, Linet, Linnet, Linnetta, Lynette, Lynnet

Linnea *Scan.* "Lime or linden tree" is the meaning given by most sources, but an informal network of people named Linnea trace the name to a mountain flower growing in northern climates that botanist Carl Linnaeus named for himself. A popular series of children's books by Christian Bjork featuring a character named Linnea has given the name greater exposure.

Linea, Linnaea, Lynea, Lynnea

Lisa Diminutive of **Elizabeth** (*Heb.* "Pledged to God"). Used in numbers only since the 1950s, and reached the top 10 in the United States in the 1970s.

Leesa, Leeza, Liesa, Lise, Liseta, Lisetta

Lissa Diminutive of **Melissa** (*Gk.* "Bee"). May also be considered a variation of **Lisa**. Unusual.

Livia Diminutive of **Olivia** (*Lat.* "Olive"). As Olivia has become trendy, this shortened version may also see more use.

Livija, Livvy, Livy, Livya, Lyvia

Liza Diminutive of **Elizabeth** and more particularly of **Eliza**. The vogue for **Lisa** gave Liza some reflected popularity, but the immense fame of entertainer Liza Minnelli must account for a great deal of its use.

Liz, Lizette, Lyza

Lois Variation of **Louise** (*OG.* "Renowned in battle," though some sources suggest Greek for "better"). Also, surprisingly enough, a biblical name. Use peaked early in the 20th century.

Lola Diminutive of **Dolores** (*Sp.* "Sorrows"). The most famous Lola has been the 19th-century courtesan Lola Montez, which has given the name a slightly racy aura. It is fairly well used regardless.

   Loela, Lolla

Lolita Diminutive of **Lola** (*Sp.* "Sorrows"). Made famous by Vladimir Nabokov's 1958 novel about a 12-year-old nymphet and her much older admirer, Humbert Humbert.

Lorenza (*Fem.* **Lorenzo**) *Lat.* "From Laurentium." Very unusual in English-speaking countries, being primarily an Italian name.

   Laurenca, Laurenza

Loretta Diminutive of **Laura** (*Lat.* "Laurel"). A name that cropped up with the 19th-century taste for elaboration and became famous with actress Loretta Young.

   Laretta, Lauretta, Laurette

Lori Diminutive of **Laura** (*Lat.* "Laurel"). This is a modern spelling and was very popular in the 1960s. The rage for the "-i" ending on names has diminished considerably since then.

   Loree, Lorri

Lorna *Scot.* Place name converted into a female name for the 19th-century romantic novel *Lorna Doone*. Used occasionally, but to most North Americans, it is probably the name of a cookie.

   Lorrna

Lorraine *Fr.* "From Lorraine." Lorraine is an area in eastern
France, but this is not just your average place name: It was
often used for Joan of Arc (who was from Lorraine). It can
also be considered an elaboration of **Lora.** Was well used
from the 1930s, and its vogue peaked in the 1940s in the
United States.

> Laraine, Larayne, Laurraine, Lerayne, Lorain,
> Loraine, Lorine, Lorrayne

Lottie Diminutive of **Charlotte** (*Fr.* "Little, womanly"). Mostly
19th-century use.

> Lotta, Lotte, Lotty

Lou Diminutive of **Louise.** Used mostly in the United States,
and in combined forms such as **Louann, Mary Lou,** and
Louella.

> Louanne, Louella, Lu, Loulou

Louise (*Fem.* **Louis**) *OG.* "Renowned in battle." Actually a
French (and more euphonious) version of **Ludwig. Louisa**
was the preferred form in the 18th and 19th centuries,
eclipsed by Louise at the turn of the 20th century.

> Aloisa, Aloysia, Eloisa, Eloise, Heloisa, Heloise,
> Lois, Lou, Louisa, Louisetta, Louisette,
> Louisiana, Louisiane, Louisina, Louisine, Lovisa,
> Ludovica, Luisa, Luise, Lula, Lulita, Lulu

Lucia *It.* Variant of **Lucy** (*Lat.* "Light"). Uncommon form in
English-speaking countries.

Lucille *Fr.* Variant of **Lucy** (*Lat.* "Light"). As **Lucilla,** used by
the Romans and revived in the 19th century. Lucille came
into use at the turn of the 20th century, and its considerable popularity (roughly 1940–1960) seems to have been
inspired by comedienne Lucille Ball.

> **Lucila, Lucile, Lucilla**

Lucinda Variation of **Lucy** (*Lat.* "Light"). Popular along with
the other "-inda" names of the 18th century (**Clarinda,
Belinda**) and boosted by the fondness for **Lucille.**

> **Cindy, Lusinda**

Lucretia *Lat.* Clan name of uncertain meaning, though some
sources suggest "wealth."

> **Lucrece, Lucrecia, Lucrezia**

Lucy *Lat.* "Light." The vernacular form of **Lucia.** More widely
used in modern times, peaking in the United States at the
turn of the 20th century. Lucy in Charles Schulz's much-
loved *Peanuts* comic strip is the prototypical bossy little
girl. For a pretty name with few negative connotations, it is
surprisingly ignored in the United States.

> **Lou, Lu, Luce, Lucetta, Luci, Lucia, Lucie,
> Lucienne, Lucile, Lucilla, Lucille, Lucina,
> Lucinda, Lucine, Lucita, Lusita, Luz**

Luella *OE.* Combination of **Louise** (*OG.* "Renowned in battle")
and **Ella** (*OG.* "All").

> **Louella, Lula, Lulu**

Lupe *Sp.* Allusion to the Virgin Mary as she miraculously appeared to a peasant boy in Guadalupe, Mexico.
> Lupelina

Luz *Sp.* "Light." Another name for the Virgin Mary: Santa María de Luz.
> Lucita, Lusita

Lydia *Gk.* "From Lydia." Lydia was an area of Asia famous for its two rich kings, Midas and Croesus. The name (biblical in origin) was used heavily in the 18th and 19th centuries, less so in the 20th.
> Lidia, Lyda, Lydie

Lynette *Welsh.* "Idol." Though it looks like a modern elaboration of **Lynn**, this is actually a French version of the Welsh **Eiluned** and was popularized by the English poet Tennyson. However, its use has certainly depended on the appeal of Lynn.
> Linett, Linette, Lynetta

Lynn Diminutive of **Linda** (*Sp.* "Pretty"). Along with its variations, the name is so popular as to virtually swamp its source. Most used in the 20th century.
> Lin, Linn, Linnell, Lyn, Lyndell, Lynelle, Lynette

Mabel Diminutive of **Amabel** (*Lat.* "Lovable"). Very popular at the turn of the 20th century but uncommon now.

> **Amabel, Mab, Mabelle, Mable**

Mackenzie *Ir. Gael.* "Son of the wise ruler." Transferred last name and quite trendy for girls today.

> **MacKensie, McKensie, McKenzie**

Macy *OF.* Place name: "Matthew's estate." Another transferred last name that may sound feminine; well used for girls.

> **Macey**

Madeline *Gk.* Place name: Magdala was a town on the Sea of Galilee, the home of Saint Mary Magdalen, who Jesus healed and who was present at his crucifixion. **Magdalen** was the common form in the Middle Ages, but the "g" was dropped, leaving Madeline as the standard form. The French version, **Madeleine,** became more popular in the 1930s, but the name, pretty as it is, has never been a standard.

> **Madalaina, Maddie, Madeleine, Magdalen, Malina, Maude**

Madison *OE.* "Son of the mighty warrior." Another obscure masculine name that has crossed over into fashionable use

for girls. It has been in the top 10 names for American girls
since 1997.

   Maddie, Madisen, Madisson

Maggie Diminutive of **Margaret** (*Gk.* "Pearl"). Used as an
   independent name in the late 19th century.

   Magali, Maggey, Maggy, Maguy

Mahala *Heb.* "Tender affection." Old Testament name that
   was well used in the 19th century.

   Mahalia, Mehalia

Maia *Gk.* "Mother." In Greek myth, a nymph who became
   mother of Hermes; also the Roman goddess of the springtime, for whom the month of May is named.

   Maaja, Maja, May, Maya, Mya

Maisie Diminutive of **Margaret** (*Gk.* "Pearl"). Originally a
   Scottish variation by way of **Margery**, it became more
   widespread early in the 20th century.

   Maisey, Maisy

Malka *Heb.* "Queen."

   Malke, Milka

Mallory *OF.* "Unhappy, unlucky." Literally, *malheureux.*

   Mallary, Malory

Mamie Diminutive of **Margaret** (*Gk.* "Pearl") or **Mary** (*Heb.*
   "Bitter").

   Maime, Mame

Mandisa *South African.* "Sweet."

Mandy Diminutive of **Amanda** (*Lat.* "Much-loved").
> **Manda, Mandie**

Mansi *Hopi.* "Plucked flower."

Manuela (*Fem.* **Emmanuel**) *Sp.* from *Heb.* "The Lord is among us."
> **Manuelita**

Mara *Heb.* "Bitter." In the Old Testament, Naomi says, "Call me Mara, for the Almighty has dealt very bitterly with me." This is widely considered to be the root of that all-time favorite, **Mary.**
> **Maraline, Mari, Marra**

Marcella (*Fem.* **Marcellus**) *Lat.* "Warlike." First cropped up at the turn of the 20th century. Very unusual.
> **Marcela, Marcelle, Marcellina, Marcie, Marcy, Marsella**

Marcia (*Fem.* **Mark**) *Lat.* "Warlike." Used in Imperial Rome and not revived until the late 19th century. It gradually became a great favorite in the middle of the 20th century but was passé by the 1970s.
> **Marci, Marsha, Marsia, Martia**

Margaret *Gk.* "Pearl." One of the standard female names of the Western world. In the Middle Ages the virgin martyr Saint Margaret (swallowed by a dragon) was hugely popular, keeping the name current. It has been neck and neck with **Mary** from the 17th century until the 1970s, when more novel names started moving to the forefront.

Greta, Gretchen, Gretel, Maggy, Mairead, Maisie,
Marcheta, Margalit, Margarethe, Margarita,
Margerie, Margisia, Margrid, Marguerite,
Marjorey, Marquetta, Meg, Meta, Peggy, Rita

Margo *Fr.* Diminutive of **Margaret**.

Margaux, Margot

Marguerite *Fr.* Variant of **Margaret**. Also botanical, the
French name for a daisy, and popular at the same time
(late 19th century to mid-20th) as that flower name.

Margarite, Margherita, Marguerita

Maria *Lat.* Variant of **Mary** (*Heb.* "Bitter"). Launched in
English-speaking countries in the 18th century as a wel-
come alternative to the all-too-common Mary. Faded after
some two hundred years, but revived in the middle of the
20th century, particularly after the popularity of *West Side
Story,* with its famous ballad "Maria." This version is now
slightly more popular than the Anglophone Mary.

Mariah, Marie, Marja, Marya

Marian *Fr.* Combination of **Mary** (*Heb.* "Bitter") and
Ann (*Heb.* "Grace"). Variant of **Mary**. Actually an anglicization of **Marion**. Common in the Middle Ages and revived
in the early Victorian era when medieval history was very
popular.

Mariana, Mariane, Marion

Marianne *Fr.* Combination of **Marie** (*Heb.* "Bitter") and
Anne (*Heb.* "Grace"). Like **Annemarie**, combines the

names of the Virgin Mary and her mother, thus appealing powerfully to Catholic families. In English-speaking countries **Mary Ann** is the standard form.

> Mariana, Mariane, Maryann

Maribel Combination of **Mary** (*Heb.* "Bitter") and **Belle** (*Fr.* "Beautiful"). This is a modern name.

> Maribelle, Meribel

Marie *Fr.* Variation of **Mary** (*Heb.* "Bitter"). Also the earliest English spelling of the name, revived in the 19th century, and in the 1970s nearly as popular as Mary.

> Maree

Marilyn Diminutive of **Mary** (*Heb.* "Bitter"). Possibly also a combination of **Mary** and **Ellen** (*Gk.* "Light"). In any case, a modern name.

> Maralin, Marilynne, Marrilyn, Marylyn

Marina *Lat.* "From the sea," as in "marine." In the distant mists of time, possibly related to the Latin god of war, Mars.

> Marinna, Marna

Maris *Lat.* "Of the sea." Comes from the phrase *stella maris,* or "star of the sea," which refers to the Virgin Mary.

> Marisa, Marise, Marissa

Marisol Combination of **Mary** (*Heb.* "Bitter") and **sol** (*Sp.* "Sun"). A modern name particularly favored in Puerto Rico.

Marjorie Variant of **Margery**, diminutive of **Margaret** (*Gk.* "Pearl"). Imported to England in the 12th century as

Margery and steadily used there until a late 19th-century revival that lasted into the 1930s. This is currently the most common form.

Marge, Margery, Margie, Marjory

Marlene Combination of **Mary** (*Heb.* "Bitter") and **Magdalene** (*Gk.* "From Magdala"). Marlene Dietrich introduced the name in the 1920s, and it was widespread by the 1940s but is now rare.

Marla, Marlane, Marleen, Marley, Marlynne

Martha *Aramaic.* "Lady." In the New Testament, Martha is the woman who bustles around, resentfully getting dinner ready while her sister, Mary, listens to Jesus. The name has been very widely used since the Puritans revived it, though it is less common since the 1960s.

Marfa, Marta, Marthe, Marthena, Martita, Mattie

Martina (*Fem.* **Martin**) *Lat.* "Warlike."

Marta, Martine

Mary *Heb.* "Bitter, bitterness" or "rebellious." Mary is the Greek version of **Miriam**. Although until the Middle Ages it was considered too sacred to use, it gradually became the most common female name. The numerous variants, both English and foreign, cropped up as a result of the name's great popularity. Ironically, the name once thought of as completely commonplace is now quite unusual among young children.

Malia, Mamie, Manette, Mara, Marabel, Marella, Maria, Marian, Mariann, Marianna, Marie,

Mariel, Marilin, Marilla, Marita, Marja, Marla, Masha, Maura, May, Mimi, Minnie, Miriam, Mitzi, Moira, Mollie, Morag, Polly

Matilda *OG.* "Battle-mighty." William the Conqueror's wife took the name to Britain in the 11th century, when it was pronounced "Maud." Most parents know it only from the famous Australian song "Waltzing Matilda."

Mafalda, Mathilda, Mathilde, Maud, Maude, Tilda, Tillie

Maud Variation of **Matilda**. Although a common enough name after the Middle Ages, its period of real popularity was 1840 to 1910.

Maude, Maudie

Maureen *Ir.* Variant of **Mary** (*Heb.* "Bitter"). Popular in the baby boom era, but to today's parents, this is a name for a previous generation.

Maura, Maurine, Moira

Maxine *Lat.* "Greatest." A modern name that had its moment from the fifties through the seventies.

Massima, Maxence, Maxene

May Several possible sources: a medieval form of **Matthew** (Mayhew), a nickname form of **Mary**, or an anglicization of **Maia**. It was very fashionable in the United States in the 1870s, some fifty years before month names (**April** and **June**) became current.

Mae, Maia, Maj, Maya

Megan *Welsh.* Diminutive of **Margaret** (*Gk.* "Pearl"). Fairly
widespread in the 20th century, and surged into popularity in
the early 1990s, when it hit the top 10 in the United States.
> **Meaghan, Meg, Meghan**

Melanie *Gk.* "Black, dark skinned." Uncommon until the
publication of *Gone with the Wind,* whose Melanie Wilkes
launched it into fashion.
> **Mel, Mela, Melaina, Melaine, Melaney**

Melinda *Lat.* "Honey." Names ending in "-inda" (**Belinda,
Clarinda**) were very fashionable in the 18th century, when
this name was coined. It became more widespread in the
19th century but is still far from common.
> **Linda, Malina, Malinda**

Melissa *Gk.* "Bee." A name that existed in ancient Greece and
occurred steadily through the 19th century but had no real
vogue in English-speaking countries until the 1970s. Now
somewhat neglected.
> **Lissa, Mel, Melicent, Melisande, Melisse,
> Mellisa, Missy**

Melody *Gk.* "Song." Though it occurred as early as the 13th
century, common usage didn't develop until the 1940s,
and it didn't endure.
> **Melodia, Melodie**

Mercedes *Sp.* "Mercies." Refers to Santa Maria de las
Mercedes, or Our Lady of the Mercies. Mostly Catholic use.
> **Merced, Mercede, Mercedez**

Mercy *ME.* "Mercy." One of the names of virtues so popular among the Puritans.

> **Merci, Mercie**

Meredith *Old Welsh.* "Great ruler." Occasionally used for boys, especially in Wales. Elsewhere a girl's name used with some frequency.

> **Meradith, Meridith**

Merle *Fr.* "Blackbird." Use probably inspired by actress Merle Oberon, whose middle name it was.

> **Merla, Meryl**

Merry *OE.* "Lighthearted, happy." Also diminutive of **Meredith** and **Mercy.** May also be considered a variant of its homonym, **Mary.**

> **Merrie, Merrilee**

Meryl Variant of **Muriel** via **Meriel.** Strictly a 20th-century name, which in the United States is strongly associated with actress Meryl Streep.

> **Merel, Merrell, Merrill, Meryle**

Mia *It.* "Mine."

> **Mea, Meya**

Michaela (*Fem. Michael*) *Heb.* "Who is like the Lord?" The most common feminine form of Michael is the French **Michelle,** but Michaela gained ground briefly in the 1990s.

> **Macaela, Micaela, Michaelina, Mickie, Miguela, Miguelita, Mikaela**

Michelle (*Fr. Fem.* **Michael**) *Fr.* Variation of *Heb.* "Who is like the Lord?" Spelled with one or two l's, fashionable right from its 1940s appearance in English-speaking countries. The Beatles' famous song "Michelle" gave the name even more of a boost, putting it on some top 10 lists in the 1970s. Now past its prime.

> Mechelle, Michaella, Michal, Michele, Micheline, Mickie, Miguela

Michiko *Jap.* "The righteous way."

> Michee, Michi

Milagros *Sp.* "Miracles."

> Mila, Milagritos, Miligrosa

Mildred *OE.* "Gentle strength." An Anglo-Saxon name that was revived in the 17th century, but its real popularity came in the United States from 1900 to 1930. By the time of the 1945 film *Mildred Pierce,* it was already slightly dated.

> Mildrid, Millie, Milly

Millicent *OG.* "Highborn power." Norman name that has been used mostly in Britain. At its most fashionable around 1900 but never a standard.

> Mel, Melicent, Melisande, Mellicent, Mellie, Millie

Mimi Diminutive of **Mary**, **Miriam**, and so forth. First used by parents after the appearance of Puccini's famous opera *La Bohème,* whose tragic heroine is named Mimi.

Minerva *Lat.* Roman goddess of wisdom. Those great revivalists, the Victorians, brought it back for their daughters, but by the Jazz Age it was obsolete.

Minnie Diminutive of **Mary** and **Wilhelmina**. Enjoyed a great vogue as an independent name around the 1870s.

> **Minny**

Mira *Lat.* "Admirable." Diminutive of **Miranda** or variation of **Myra**.

> **Mirra, Myra, Myrène**

Mirabel *Lat.* "Wonderful." In this case, the "-bel" ending does not mean "beautiful," though the variations often spell it "-belle."

> **Meribel, Mirabelle**

Miranda *Lat.* "Admirable." Another name contributed to us by Shakespeare, this time directly from the Latin: He used it for the heroine of *The Tempest*. Use has been steadily slight.

> **Maranda, Mira, Mireille, Mirella, Randa, Randie**

Miriam *Heb.* Possibly "bitter" or "rebellious." This is the source of **Mary**, which is its Latin form, and its translation is not quite clear, though "bitter" is very widely accepted. Quite common for some two hundred fifty years, peaking around 1900 in the United States. Now unusual.

> **Mariam, Maryam, Meryam, Mimi**

Molly Diminutive of **Mary** (*Heb.* "Bitter"). Not Irish, in spite of the famous song "Cockles and Mussels" about Dublin's "sweet Molly Malone." The name has had long periods of disuse but has found its way into the top 100 in the United States.

Moll, Molley, Mollie

Mona *Ir. Gael.* "Aristocratic." Spread from Ireland in the mid-19th century. Never widespread but common enough not to be outlandish.

Monah, Moyna

Monica Possibly *Lat.* "Adviser" or "nun." Established by Saint Monica, the mother of Saint Augustine, and favored by Catholic families.

Mona, Monicka, Monika, Monique

Morgan Different sources give different meanings, including Welsh for "great and bright" and *OE.* for "bright or white sea dweller." Quite well used for girls in the United States.

Morgana, Morgane

Moriah *Heb.* "The Lord is my teacher." May also be arrived at as a variant of **Maria, Mariah,** and **Mary.**

Moraia, Moraiah

Mouna *Arab.* "Wish, desire."

Mounia, Muna, Munira

Muriel *Ir. Gael.* "Sea bright." Some names, such as this one, seem rooted in a certain period (in this case, the first half of the 20th century), but Muriel actually dates back to the

Middle Ages. Perhaps the children of the 21st century will eventually find it nostalgic enough to use for *their* children.

Merial, Murial, Murielle

Myra (*Fem.* **Myron**) *Lat.* "Scented oil." Literary name coined in the early 17th century, but real-life use dates from the 19th century.

Maira, Mira, Myree

Myrna *Ir. Gael.* "Tender, beloved." The era of the name's popularity, the 1930s and 1940s, spans the career of actress Myrna Loy.

Meirna, Mirna

Nabila *Arab.* "Highborn."

Nabeela

Nadia *Rus.* "Hope." **Nada** appeared in English-speaking countries at the turn of the 20th century, but Nadia did not take root until the 1960s. Though not outlandish, it has a pleasantly foreign sound.

Nada, Nadine, Nadiya, Nadja, Nadya

Nancy Variant of **Ann** (*Heb.* "Grace"). Originally a nickname whose use as a given name began in the 18th century.

Took root firmly and was very popular in the United States in the middle of the 20th century.

>Nance, Nancee, Nanci, Nancie, Nannie, Nanny, Nansey

Naomi *Heb.* "Pleasant." Old Testament name; the mother-in-law of Ruth, who, after her sons died, said, "Do not call me Naomi, call me Mara, for the Almighty has dealt very bitterly with me." Naomi came into English-speaking use not with the Puritan revival of biblical names but in the 18th century.

>Naoma, Noémi, Noémie

Nastasia *Gk.* "Resurrection." Diminutive of **Anastasia**.

>Nastassia, Nastassja

Natalie *Lat.* "Birth day." More specifically, the Lord's birthday, or Christmas. This is probably the most common of all the Christmas names and certainly the only one that is used for babies born at other times of the year (unlike **Noel**). It has become quite fashionable in recent years.

>Natalee, Natalia, Natalya, Natasha, Nathalie, Natividad, Talia, Tasha

Nell Diminutive of **Helen** and **Eleanor** (*Gk.* "Light"). Used sparingly as an independent name, though some of its variants such as **Nellie** have had periods of popularity.

>Nella, Nellie, Nelly

Nettie Diminutive of "-ette" names such as **Henrietta** or

Nanette. Use as an independent name mostly around the turn of the 20th century.

Netta, Netty

Nicole (*Fem.* **Nicholas**) *Gk.* "Victory of the people." **Nicola,** the Italian form, is more common in Britain (though its vogue peaked there in the 1970s). This French version has been more popular in other English-speaking countries, reaching the top 10 in the United States in the 1980s.

Cola, Colette, Cosetta, Nichola, Nicholette, Nicholle, Nicia, Nicki, Nickola, Nicky, Nico, Nicola, Nicoleen, Nicolette, Nicolle, Nika, Niki, Nikki, Nychole

Nina *Sp.* "Girl." Diminutive of **Ann** (*Heb.* "Grace"). History buffs will remember that Nina was the name of one of Christopher Columbus's three ships. The name is rather uncommon.

Neina, Nenna, Nineta, Ninette, Ninochka, Ninon

Noel *Fr.* "Christmas." Though used since the Middle Ages for both boys and girls, it is more common for the latter.

Noela, Noelene, Noella, Noelle, Nowell

Nona *Lat.* "Ninth." Although it was originally used for a family's ninth baby, it would hardly have survived to this day if parents had not been willing to overlook its meaning.

Nonah, Noni, Nonie, Nonna, Nonnah

Nora Diminutive of **Eleanor** (*Gk.* "Light") and **Honora** (*Lat.* "Woman of honor"). Used independently, especially for the half century around 1900. Well-read parents will remember Nora as the heroine of Ibsen's *A Doll's House;* she sets a discouraging precedent, however.

Norah, Norella, Norelle

Noreen *Ir.* Diminutive of **Nora.** Originated in Ireland.

Norene, Norina, Norine

Norma *Lat.* "Pattern." From the same root that gave us "normal" or "the norm." Launched by Bellini's 1831 opera of the same name and boosted in the 1920s by popular actress Norma Shearer. Out of fashion for the last couple of generations.

Norm, Normie, Normina

Nur *Arab.* "Light." The Arabic name adopted by the former queen of Jordan, an American woman known as Lisa Halaby until she married the king.

Noor, Nour

Odessa *Gk.* "Long voyage." As in "odyssey," more specifically Homer's epic poem about the wandering Odysseus.

Odissa, Odyssa, Odyssia

Odette *Fr.* from *Ger.* "Wealthy." In the famous ballet *Swan Lake,* the same ballerina usually dances as both Odette, the good swan, and Odile, the evil black swan.

>   **Odetta**

Odile *Fr.* Variant of **Otthild** (*OG.* "Prospers in battle"). Related to **Odette** and also to **Odelia.** For balletomanes, the malevolent alter ego of Odette.

Olga *Rus.* "Holy." The Russian form of **Helga,** it is perhaps more common than Helga in English-speaking countries. The name was favored in the ill-fated Russian imperial family.

>   **Elga, Helga, Ola**

Oliana *Polynesian.* "Oleander."

>   **Oleana, Olianna**

Olinda *Lat.* "Scented."

Olivia *Lat.* "Olive tree." The most common form of the name today, though **Olive** had a flurry of popularity with other nature names at the turn of the 20th century. This form, though, is speeding up popularity charts.

>   **Livia, Livvy, Olia, Oliva, Olive, Olivet, Ollie, Olva**

Olympia *Gk.* "From Mount Olympus," the home of the gods. Slightly more common in Europe.

>   **Olimpia, Olimpiana, Olypme, Olympie**

Oma *Arab.* "Leader." Infrequent use.

Ondine *Lat.* "Little wave." In mythology, Undine is the spirit of the waters.

>   **Ondina, Ondyne, Undine**

Oneida *Native American.* "Long awaited." In the United States, probably most familiar as a brand of silverware that was originally manufactured by a utopian colony disbanded in the 19th century because its residents practiced polygamy.

> Onida, Onyda

Onella *Gk.* "Light."

Onora Variant of **Honoria** (*Lat.* "Honor").

> Onnora, Onoria, Onorine

Oona *Ir.* Variant of **Una** (*Lat.* "Unity").

> Oonagh, Una

Opal *Sanskrit.* "Gem." One of the less common of the jewel names.

> Opalina, Opaline

Ophelia *Gk.* "Help." Most famously, the young girl in *Hamlet* who goes mad. Mostly used in the late 19th century, but its connotations are far from happy.

> Ofelia, Ophélie, Ophilia

Ora *Lat.* "Prayer." Homonym for **Aura**, which means "gold" or "breeze."

> Orabel, Orabelle

Oralee *Heb.* "My light."

> Orali, Oralit, Orlee

Oriana *Lat.* "Dawning." From the same root as **Aurora**.

> Oria, Oriane, Orianna

Orpah *Heb.* "A fawn." Old Testament name rarely used.
Talk show star Oprah Winfrey's unusual name is the result
of a misspelling of this name.

> Ophrah, Oprah, Orpa

Orquidea *Sp.* "Orchid."

Orsa Variation of **Ursula** (*Lat.* "Bear").

> Orsalina, Orsola, Ursa

Otthild *OG.* "Prospers in battle." **Odile** is perhaps the most
common form.

> Odile, Ottilie, Ottoline, Otylia

Page *Fr.* A young boy in training as a personal assistant to a
knight. Usually a transferred surname, possibly indicating
an ancestor who was a page. Use as a girl's name is quite
recent.

> Padget, Paget, Paige

Paloma *Sp.* "Dove."

> Palometa, Palomita

Pamela *Gk.* "All honey." Literary name coined at the end of
the 16th century, growing gradually more common until a
distinct vogue in the 1950s and 1960s.

> Pam, Pamelia, Pamella, Pammie

Pandora *Gk.* "All gifted." In Greek mythology Pandora was
the first woman, endowed with gifts by all the gods. She
is famous for the box that was her dowry; it contained all
the world's evils, which flew out when the box was opened.
One of the more common of the Greek names in English-
speaking countries but still highly unusual.
    Dora, Panndora

Paquita *Sp.* Diminutive of **Frances** (*Lat.* "From France") via
Paco.

Paris Place name: the capital city of France. Almost unknown
until the early 2000s, when usage increased strikingly.
Paris Hilton may be responsible.
    Parris, Parrish

Pat Diminutive of **Patricia.** Used as an independent name but
neglected with the recent leaning toward the nostalgic and
elaborate.

Patience Virtue name. One of the more popular of the 16th-
century names, though eclipsed in the 20th century by
Faith and **Hope.**
    Paciencia, Pazienza

Patricia (*Fem.* **Patrick**) *Lat.* "Noble, patrician." Obscure until
it was used for one of Queen Victoria's granddaughters,
which launched its enormous popularity for close to fifty
years. It has now returned to near neglect.
    **Pat, Patrice, Patrizia, Patsy, Pattee, Patti, Pattie,
Tricia, Trish, Trisha**

Paula (*Fem.* **Paul**) *Lat.* "Small." Roman name that cropped up in English-speaking countries in this century and was rather well used in the baby boom era.

> Paola, Paolina, Paule, Pauletta, Paulette, Paulina, Pauline, Pavla, Pola, Polina, Pollie, Polly

Paz *Sp.* "Peace."

Pearl *Lat.* "Pearl." Probably the most common of the jewel names, though of course it is not a gemstone. The Greek form, **Margaret,** is far more widespread and has been used for centuries, while Pearl only appeared in the late Victorian era.

> Pearla, Pearle, Pearleen, Pearlette, Pearline

Peggy Diminutive of **Margaret** (*Gk.* "Pearl"). Used as an independent name since the 18th century, and parents who choose it today probably do so without thinking of Margaret.

> Peg, Pegeen, Peggie

Penelope *Gk.* "Bobbin worker." The bobbin probably refers to part of the equipment for weaving, since the Penelope of Greek myth was the wife of Odysseus. To put off the many suitors who courted her when it seemed that the wandering Odysseus must be dead, she told them she couldn't marry until she finished the tapestry she was weaving. She would work all day and unravel her work at night, hoping that her husband would come home. The

name was most popular in the middle of the 20th century
in Britain.

Pen, Penny

Penny Diminutive of **Penelope** (*Gk.* "Bobbin worker"). Given
as an independent name mostly in the 20th century.

Pepita *Sp.* Diminutive of **Joseph** (*Heb.* "Jehovah increases")
via **Pepe.**

Pepa, Peta

Petra (*Fem.* **Peter**) *Gk.* "Rock." The simplest feminization of a
name that seems to resist being feminized.

**Peta, Peterina, Petrina, Petrine, Petronela,
Petronella, Pierette, Pierrette, Pietra**

Philippa (*Fem.* **Philip**) *Gk.* "Horse lover." Another unusual
feminization, though it was used somewhat in the 19th
century.

Filipa, Filipina, Philippine, Pippa

Phoebe *Gk.* "Shining, brilliant." One of the epithets of Apollo,
the sun god, was Phoebus Apollo, referring to the fact that
he brought light. Phoebe appears in the New Testament,
but the name didn't gain ground until the 18th century. It
reached a peak in the last part of the 19th century and is
now pleasantly old-fashioned and ripe for revival.

Phebe, Pheby, Phoebey

Phyllida Variant of **Phyllis** (*Gk.* "Leafy bough"). Rare name
that appeared in the 16th century; mostly literary use.

Fillida, Phillida, Phillyda

Phyllis *Gk.* "Leafy bough." Name of a mythological woman, taken up by generations of poets to stand for the idealized country lass. The name was used increasingly through the 19th century, but it died out after the 1930s.

> Filis, Fillis, Phillis, Phyllida, Phylliss

Pia *Lat.* "Pious." More common in Europe.

Piedad *Sp.* "Piety, devotion."

Pilar *Sp.* "Pillar." An allusion to the Virgin Mary in her role as a "pillar" of the Church. Used mostly by Spanish-speaking parents.

Pippa Diminutive of **Philippa** (*Gk.* "Lover of horses"). Almost exclusively British use.

> Pippy

Polly Variant of **Molly**. Diminutive of **Mary** (*Heb.* "Bitter"). Independent name used especially in the 19th century. Never as common as Molly, for no discernible reason.

> Poll, Polley, Pollie

Portia *Lat.* Clan name, obscure meaning. The heroine of Shakespeare's *Merchant of Venice,* an enterprising woman who disguises herself as a lawyer to save her husband's life. In spite of this worthy prototype, the name is uncommon.

Prima *Lat.* "First."

> Primalia, Primetta, Primina, Priminia

Primavera *It.* "Spring." Pretty name for a spring baby.

Primrose *ME.* "First rose." The primrose does not actually

belong to the rose family, but it is one of the flowers that
blooms early in spring. A 19th-century flower name.

Primarosa, Primorosa, Primula

Priscilla *Lat.* "Ancient." New Testament name common in the
early Christian era, then revived strongly by the Puritans.
After generations of neglect, it was taken up in the 19th
century but has been scarce since the last half of the 20th
century, possibly because the most natural nickname is
"Prissy."

Cilla, Pris, Prisca, Prissy, Prysilla

Prudence *Lat.* "Caution, discretion." Virtue name most common in the 19th century after its first popularity in the 16th
and 17th centuries. Use now is mostly British.

Pru, Prudencia, Prudie, Prudy, Prue

Prunella *Lat.* "Small plum."

Prunelle

Psyche *Gk.* "Breath," and, by extension, life or soul. In
mythology Psyche was a mortal girl who Cupid loved. In
post-Freudian times someone's psyche is her innermost
soul or mind.

Queen *OE.* "Queen."
> **Queenie**

Querida *Sp.* "Dear, beloved."

Quinn *Ir. Gael.* Meaning unknown. Very common Irish last
> name occasionally transferred to first-name status, though
> less often for girls.

Rachel *Heb.* "Ewe, female sheep." In the Old Testament
> Rachel is the wife of the patriarch Jacob. Parents in the
> late 1960s and 1970s used it in great numbers. Still very
> popular into the 1990s, now less of a favorite.
>
> **Rachael, Rachele, Rachelle, Rae, Rahel, Raquel,
> Ray**

Rae Diminutive of **Rachel** (*Heb.* "Ewe"). Used independently
> in modern times.
>
> **Ray, Raye**

Ramona (*Fem.* **Raymond**) *Sp.* "Wise guardian." A 19th-
> century historical novel of the same title was immensely

successful and brought the name to wide attention, but it is scarce now.

Mona, Romona

Rani *Sanskrit.* "Queen."

Rana, Ranee, Rania

Ranita *Heb.* "Song."

Ranice, Ranit

Raphaela (*Fem.* **Raphael**) *Heb.* "God heals." Unusual feminization, though used with some frequency in Italy.

Rafaela, Rafaella

Rashida (*Fem.* **Rashid**) *Turkish.* "Righteous, rightly advised."

Rasheda, Rasheeda

Raven Name of the large black bird that is closely related to the crow. A fanciful name for a black-haired or dark-skinned baby.

Ravenne, Rayven

Rebecca *Heb.* "Joined." A prominent Old Testament name; Rebecca is the wife of Isaac and mother of Jacob and Esau. Predictably, the name was taken up by the Puritans and remained fairly common through the 19th century. Subsequent revivals (in the thirties in the United States, in the late sixties in Britain) may have been prompted by literary and cinematic use of the name, especially in the novel and film *Rebecca*.

Becca, Becka, Becky, Reba, Rebekah, Riva, Rivah, Rivka, Rivkah

Regina *Lat.* "Queen." Cropped up at the end of the Victorian era, possibly encouraged by the fact that Her Majesty was often known as Victoria Regina. It may also be used as an allusion to the Virgin Mary, Regina Coelis ("Queen of the Heavens").

> Gina, Raina, Raine, Régine, Reine

Remedios *Sp.* "Help, remedy." Currently popular in South America.

Remy *Fr.* "From Rheims." Champagne and the fine brandies made from champagne are the principal products of Rheims, a town in central France.

> Remi, Remie

Rena *Heb.* "Melody," or diminutive of **Irene** (*Gk.* "Peace").

> Reena, Rina

Renée *Fr.* "Reborn." The French form of **Renata**, more common (though not really widespread) in modern times.

> Ranae, Renae, Renate, René, Renita

Rhea *Gk.* "Earth." In Greek myth, Rhea was an earth mother who bore Zeus, Demeter, Hera, and Poseidon, among other gods.

> Rea, Rhia, Ria

Rhoda *Gk.* "Rose"; *Lat.* "From Rhodes." Rhodes is a Greek island originally named for its roses. The name is found in the New Testament and was used mostly in the 18th and 19th centuries.

> Rhodia, Rhodie, Rhody

Rhona *ONorse.* "Rough island." A form of **Rona** more common in Britain.

> **Rhona, Roana**

Rhonda Welsh place name: The Rhondda Valley is a significant landmark in southern Wales, named for the river that runs through it. (In Welsh, the name means "noisy.")

> **Rhonnda, Ronda**

Rickie Diminutive of **Frederica** (*OG.* "Peaceful ruler"). Also possibly a feminine version of **Richard** and certainly more popular than the longer forms. Occurred most often in the middle of the 20th century.

> **Rica, Ricki, Rickie, Rikki**

Rima *Arab.* "Antelope."

Risa *Lat.* "Laughter." A pretty name but very unusual in English-speaking countries.

> **Riesa, Rise, Rysa**

Rita Diminutive of **Margaret** (*Gk.* "Pearl"). Comes via the Spanish form, **Margarita**. First used on its own some hundred years ago and quite popular for fifty years.

> **Reeta, Reita**

Riva Variation of **Rebecca** (*Heb.* "Joined"). Also possibly from the French for "shore," but the Jewish families who use it most often probably have the Old Testament associations in mind.

> **Reeva, Rivka, Rivke**

Roberta (*Fem. Robert*) *OE.* "Bright fame." Rather widespread between its introduction in the late 19th century and its fall from favor some eighty years later.

> Berta, Bertie, Bobbette, Bobbie, Bobine, Robby, Robin, Robyn

Robin Diminutive of **Robert** (*OE.* "Bright fame"). Originally a boy's nickname (as in Winnie the Pooh's friend Christopher Robin), but it was appropriated for girls in increasing numbers starting in the middle of the 20th century. Now out of fashion for both sexes.

> Robbin, Robyn

Rochelle *Fr.* Place name: "little rock." Enthusiastically used as a first name starting in the 1940s but rare now.

> Rochella, Roshelle

Rohana *Sanskrit.* "Sandalwood."

> Rohanna

Roma *It.* Place name: the capital city, Rome. Rather widely used since it first appeared in the late 19th century, though it never approached the popularity of **Florence.**

> Romelle, Romola

Rona *ONorse.* "Rough island." In Britain, used interchangeably with **Rhona.** Both versions cropped up at the turn of the 20th century and have occurred steadily without ever being fashionable.

> Rhona, Ronella, Ronna

Rosabel Combination of **Rose** and **Belle** that appeared in the mid-19th century.

    Rosabella, Rosabelle

Rosalie *Fr.* Possibly "rose garden." Mostly 19th-century use.

    Rosalee, Rosalia, Rosalina

Rosalind *Sp.* "Pretty rose" is the most common interpretation, though the name was actually coined in 16th-century Britain. Used since the mid-19th century, with a surge in the middle of the 20th century.

    Rosalin, Rosaline, Rosalyn, Roselinde, Roslyn, Roz

Rosamond *OG.* "Renowned protector." Also translatable (from the Latin) as "rose of the world." More popular in the 19th century than it is today.

    Ros, Rosamonde, Rosamund, Rosamunda

Rose *Lat.* Flower name. Scholars actually trace the name to an Old German name meaning something like "renown," but the flower meaning has had much more currency, particularly given the Christian symbolic meaning of the rose. (The "rosa mystica" is the Virgin Mary.) Its popularity peaked at the turn of the 20th century.

    Rhoda, Rhodia, Rhody, Rosa, Rosalie, Rosaria, Rosie, Rosina, Rosita

Roseanne Combination of **Rose** and **Anne.** The pairing of the two names appeared in the 18th century, and various forms have drifted in and out of popularity.

    Rosanagh, Rosanna, Rosanne, Rozanne

Rosemary *Lat.* "Dew of the sea" is the correct meaning, though the name gained great currency with the flower name fad of the late 19th century. The fact that most parents read it as a combination of **Rose** and **Mary** (both already popular, and with strong religious resonance for Catholics) couldn't have hurt.

Rosemaria, Rosemarie, Rosmarie

Rowena *Welsh.* "Slender and fair." This meaning is an approximation. The name was actually brought to public notice by novelist Sir Walter Scott with his immensely popular *Ivanhoe* in the early 19th century.

Roweena, Roweina, Rowina

Roxanne *Per.* "Dawn." The wife of Alexander the Great was named Roxane.

Oksana, Roxanna, Roxy, Ruksana, Ruxana

Ruby Jewel name. Launched in the 1870s with other jewel names but passé by the mid-20th century.

Rubee, Rubetta, Rubey, Rubi, Rubia, Rubina

Ruth *Heb.* "Friend, companion." The Old Testament Book of Ruth is about the widowed Moabite woman who refuses to leave her Hebrew mother-in-law, Naomi, and says, "Whither thou goest, I will go." The name has been consistently used ever since the 17th century, peaking at the turn of the 20th century.

Ruthe, Ruthie

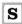

Saba *Gk.* "From Sheba"; *Arab.* "Morning." The queen of Sheba is mentioned in the Old Testament as having been hugely rich and very ostentatious.
   Sabah, Sheba, Shebah

Sabina *Lat.* "Sabine." The Sabines were a tribe living in central Italy around the time that Romulus and Remus established the city of Rome. In an effort to provide wives for the citizens of Rome, Romulus arranged the mass kidnapping of the Sabine women, which came to be known (and frequently portrayed in art and literature) as the "Rape of the Sabines." The name was used among the ancient Romans and in English-speaking countries after the 17th century.
   Sabine, Sabyna

Sabra Origin disputed: may be *Heb.* for "to rest," or possibly "cactus." It is now used as a term for a native-born Israeli.
   Sabrah, Sabrette, Sebra

Sabrina *Lat.* Place name: the Latin term for the Severn River in England. Though Milton (among others) writes about a woman named Sabrina, she appeared most vividly in modern culture as *Sabrina Fair* in the play and movie. The name was used in the 19th century and cropped up again in the last part of the 20th century.
   Brina, Sabrinna

Sachi *Jap.* "Child of joy."

    Sachiko

Sadie Diminutive of **Sarah** (*Heb.* "Princess"). Use as an independent name occurred mostly at the turn of the 20th century.

    Sada, Sydelle

Saffron Flower name: Saffron refers to a substance (the dried stamens of saffron crocuses) used as a spice in Mediterranean and other Southern cuisines.

    Saffran, Saffren, Saffronia, Saphron

Salimah *Arab.* "Healthy, sound."

    Salima, Selima

Samala *Heb.* "Requested of God."

    Samale, Sammala

Samantha (*Fem. Samuel*) *Heb.* "Told by God." Occasionally used in the 17th to 19th centuries but truly popular in the 1960s and 1970s, possibly triggered by the TV series *Bewitched*. Also popular now, having been a top 10 choice since 1988.

    Sam, Sami, Sammantha

Sandra Diminutive of **Alexandra** (*Gk.* "Defender of mankind") via *It.* **Alessandra**. Popular in the middle of the 20th century, but today's parents are more inclined to prefer the full four syllables of the original name.

    Sandie, Sandria, Sandrine, Sandy, Saundra,
    Sohndra, Sondra

Sarah *Heb.* "Princess." In the Old Testament, the wife of the patriarch Abraham. Came into vogue with other biblical names in the 16th century and was enough of a staple for four hundred years to have spawned a variety of nicknames. Sarah was in the top 10 of American girls' names since 1978 and only began to lose a little steam in 2003.

   Sadie, Sal, Sallie, Sally, Sara, Sarai

Sasha *Rus.* Feminization and diminutive of **Alexander** (*Gk.* "Man's defender"). The "-sha" ending is not necessarily feminine in Russia, and Sasha is more commonly a male nickname there.

   Sacha, Sascha

Savannah *Sp.* "Treeless." Originally familiar as a place name, as in the city in Georgia, or name of a geographical feature: a wide, treeless plain.

   Savana, Savanna, Sevanna

Scarlett *ME.* "Scarlet." Given its fame by the inimitable Scarlett O'Hara, heroine of *Gone with the Wind*.

   Scarlet, Scarletta, Scarlette

Seema *Heb.* "Precious thing, treasure."

   Cima, Cyma

Selena *Gk.* "Moon goddess." Most popular in the 19th century.

   Celie, Celina, Salena, Selene

Selima *Heb.* "Tranquil."

   Saleema, Selimah

Selma (*Fem.* **Anselm** by way of **Anselma**) *OG.* "Godly helmet."
   Sellma, Zelma

Serena *Lat.* "Tranquil, serene." Used by Roman Christians and
   periodically popular, though never in a big way.
   Serene, Serina, Serenity

Shaina *Heb.* "Beautiful."
   Shana, Shani, Shayna

Shalom *Heb.* "Peace." Not a name but a greeting to speakers
   of Hebrew. Nevertheless, adapted by some parents for its
   meaning.
   Shalome, Shalva, Shalvah, Shelom, Shilom,
   Sholome

Shaneika Modern name in the United States. Another elaboration of the popular "Sha-" prefix.
   Shanequa, Shanika, Shanta, Shantee, Sheniqua

Shannon *Ir. Gael.* "Old, ancient." The name of an important
   river, county, and airport in Ireland, used as a first name in
   the 20th and 21st centuries. Most popular among families
   with Irish roots but found infrequently in Ireland.
   Shanna, Shannen, Shanon

Shantal Variation of **Chantal** (*Fr.* Place name). Its popularity
   may be associated with other "Sha-" names rather than
   with the rather obscure French first name.
   Shanta, Shantalle, Shantay

Sharlene (*Fem.* and diminutive of **Charles**) *OG.* "Man."

Variant of **Caroline.** One of the numerous variations popular in the 1950s and 1960s.

> **Sharleen, Sharline, Sharlyne**

Sharon *Heb.* Place name: "a plain." In the Old Testament, refers to flat land at the foot of Mount Carmel. By the mid-20th century, it was quite popular in the United States.

> **Cheron, Sharen, Sharla, Sharona, Sheron**

Sheba *Heb.* "From Sheba." Also a short version of **Bathsheba** (*Heb.* "Daughter of the oath"). The queen of Sheba is mentioned in the Old Testament as having been hugely rich and very ostentatious.

> **Saba, Shebah**

Sheena Diminutive of **Sinead.** Ir. Variant of **Jane** (*Heb.* "The Lord is gracious"). Many of the "Sh" names are Gaelic versions of **Jane, Jean,** and **Joan,** which are in turn variations on that old staple, **John.**

> **Sheenah, Shena**

Sheila *Ir.* Variant of **Cecilia** (*Lat.* "Blind"). Popular in the mid-20th century in Britain and the Commonwealth.

> **Shayla, Sheela, Sheilah**

Shelley *OE.* Place name: "meadow on the ledge." Last name made famous by the poet Percy Bysshe Shelley. Use as a feminine first name seems to have been related to **Shirley.**

> **Schelley, Shellee, Shellie, Shelly**

Sherry Variant of **Cher** (*Fr.* "Dear"), **Sharon** (*Heb.* "The

plain"), or **Cheryl** (Variant of **Charlotte**, *OG*. "Man"). In the
1950s and 1960s, these three names and their variants
were all popular, giving rise to a parade of further forms,
spellings, and elaborations. Tracing the exact origin of any
of them is difficult.

> **Cheray, Cherie, Sheri**

Shifra *Heb*. "Lovely."

> **Schifra, Shifrah**

Shiri *Heb*. "My song."

> **Shira, Shirah, Shirit**

Shirley *OE*. Place name: "bright meadow." Originally a last
name, brought to immense fame and popularity as a girl's
name with the career of child star Shirley Temple. Now
widely neglected.

> **Shirely, Shirl, Shirleen**

Shoshana *Heb*. "Lily." The more common form is the anglicized **Susan** or **Susanna**.

> **Shosha, Shoshanah, Sosanna, Sosannah**

Sibyl *Gk*. "Seer, oracle." In ancient mythology, sibyls interpreted the messages from oracles devoted to particular gods,
but their legend was also taken up and Christianized, and
the name was common in the Middle Ages. Use dropped
off and was revived at the turn of the 20th century, but the
name now has a slightly dated aura.

> **Cybil, Cybill, Sibella, Sibelle, Sibilla, Sibyll,
> Sibylla, Sybil**

Sierra Place name. Sierra is Spanish for "saw" and was the
name Spanish settlers gave to the sharp, irregular peaks of
some of the Western mountains such as the Sierra Nevada
(literally, "snowy saw"). Now used from time to time as a
proper name, along with other geographical features such
as **Savannah.**

    Ciera, Cierra, Siera

Silvia Variation of **Sylvia** (*Lat.* "From the woods"). This was
the original form of the name, eclipsed by the "-y-" spelling
in the 19th century.

    Silvana, Silvanna, Silvie, Silvija, Sylvia, Sylvie

Simcha *Heb.* "Joy."

Simone (*Fem.* **Simon**) *Heb.* "Listening intently." Used outside
of France from the middle of the 20th century.

    Simeona, Simona, Simonetta, Simonette

Sinead *Ir.* Variation of **Janet** (*Fem.* **John**; *Heb.* "The Lord is
gracious"). This name and **Siobhan** are a little more common than most Gaelic names. **Sheena** is a short version
of Sinead.

    Seonaid, Shinead, Sina, Sine

Siobhan *Ir.* Variant of **Joan** (*Fem.* **John**; *Heb.* "The Lord is
gracious"). Many of the phonetic forms of this name are
probably intended as a combination of the "Sha-" prefix
and **Yvonne.**

    Shavaun, Shavon, Siobahn, Sioban

Sissy Diminutive of **Cecilia** (*Lat.* "Blind"). Also a common nickname for a sister, since this is the way a younger sibling may say that word.

> **Cecie, Cissey, Cissie**

Sonia Variation of **Sophia** (*Gk.* "Wisdom"). Used since early in the 20th century.

> **Sonja, Sonya**

Sophia *Gk.* "Wisdom." Used in English-speaking countries since the 17th century, though the French form, **Sophie**, has given it much competition in Britain. Sophia hit the top 20 American names in 2003 and is still climbing.

> **Sofia, Sofie, Sofya, Sophie, Sophy**

Speranza *It.* "Hope."

> **Esperance, Esperanza, Speranca**

Stacey *Gk.* "Resurrection." Diminutive of **Anastasia**. Most popular since the 1970s and has long since outstripped its source.

> **Stacee, Stacia, Stacie, Stacy**

Stella *Lat.* "Star." Use was mostly literary until the 19th century, when the name became fashionable. For a generation of parents brought up on classic movies, it is hard to dissociate from Marlon Brando bellowing "Stella!" in *A Streetcar Named Desire.*

> **Estella, Estelle, Estrella, Star, Stela, Stelle**

Stephanie (*Fem.* **Stephen**) *Gk.* "Crowned." Cropped up in

the 1920s and current since then. Use peaked in the top
10 in the 1990s and has since dwindled.

Estefania, Stefa, Stefania, Stefanie, Stepania

Summer *OE.* Name of the season. Largely a phenomenon
of the 1970s.

Somer, Sommers, Summers

Sunny *Eng.* Word as name: most likely to be a nickname
characterizing a child's temperament.

Sunnee, Sunnie, Sunshine

Susan *Heb.* "Lily." After 18th-century use, neglected until
a huge surge of popularity made it a top choice in the
middle years of the 20th century; thus, a name to overlook
in the 21st. Little though this form is used, it is still more
popular than either **Susanna** or **Suzanne.**

**Shoshana, Shoshanah, Sioux, Siouxsie, Sue,
Suesann, Sukey, Susana, Susanetta, Susanna,
Susannah, Susie, Susy, Suzan, Suzanne, Suze,
Suzee, Suzette, Zanna, Zanne**

Sybil Variant of Sibyl. The most common spelling of the
name, though it only became prevalent in the 19th century.

Cybill, Sibell, Sibilla, Sibyl, Sibylla Sibill

Sydney *OF.* Place name: "Saint Denis." Originally Saint Denis
would have been the name of a village, and the name
Sydney would have indicated a resident there. The name
used to be almost exclusively male. There is also a trend

toward formerly male names such as this one, which has climbed popularity charts since 1994.

Sidnee, Sidney, Sydelle, Sydnie

Sylvia *Lat.* "From the forest." The Latin form, **Silvia**, predominated for centuries, but when the name was at its most popular (from the 19th century into the 1940s), Sylvia was the spelling of choice.

Silva, Silvaine, Silvana, Silvania, Silvanna, Silvia, Sylvie

Tabitha *Aramaic.* "Gazelle." New Testament name reintroduced in the 17th-century passion for biblical names. Neglected in the 20th century until a minor revival in the 1960s.

Tabbitha, Tabetha

Tahira *Arab.* "Virginal, pure."

Talia *Heb.* "Heaven's dew." May also be a variant of **Thalia** or a derivative of **Natalie.** A pretty name but infrequently used.

Talitha *Aramaic.* "Young girl."

Taleetha, Talita

Tallulah *Choctaw Indian.* "Leaping water." Not, as one
might expect, an invented name, nor even one assumed
by its most famous bearer, actress Tallulah Bankhead. It
was a Bankhead family name and is also a place name in
Georgia.

    Tallula

Tamara *Heb.* "Palm tree." Old Testament name with a hint of
the picturesque. **Tamar** was the more common version
until the 20th century, when Tamara, the Russian form,
overtook it. Quite fashionable in the 1970s.

    Tama, Tamar, Tamarra, Tammy, Thamar

Tamika Modern name in the United States of unknown origin.

    Tameika, Tameka, Taminique, Tamiqua

Tammy Diminutive of **Tamara** (or other "Tam-" names). A
nickname that took on a life of its own in the 1950s and
1960s.

    Tami, Tamie, Tammee

Tamsin Variant of **Thomasina** (*Heb.* "Twin"). Very old name
that was revived by British parents in the middle of the
20th century.

    Tamasin, Tamsyn

Tanisha Modern name of unclear meaning. Its popularity
may stem from a contemporary fondness for three-syllable
names ending in "-a."

    Taneesha, Taniesha, Tynisha

Tanya Diminutive of **Tatiana,** an ancient Italian name.
Tana, Tahnya, Tania, Tonya

Tara *Ir. Gael.* "Rocky hill." Though Irish legends mention a
place called Tara, its real prominence came in the 1940s
when most Americans knew that Scarlett O'Hara's planta-
tion home was called Tara. This seems to have launched
the use of the name.

Tatiana *Rus.* Variant of an ancient Italian name. Has pen-
etrated the United States somewhat in recent years.
Tania, Tatianna, Tatjana

Teresa *See* **Theresa.**

Thalia *Gk.* "Blooming, in flower." In Greek legend Thalia is
one of the Three Graces.
Talia, Talley

Thea *Gk.* "Goddess." Also diminutive of **Dorothea** (*Gk.* "Gift
of God").
Tea, Theia

Thelma *Gk.* "Will." Literary name coined in the late 19th
century, at its peak in the first third of the 20th century.
Telma, Thellma

Theodora *Gk.* "Gift of God." Much less common than its
synonym, **Dorothy.** At its peak in the middle third of the
20th century but never a standard.
Dora, Feodora, Teodora, Theda, Theodosia

Theophania *Gk.* "God's appearance." Immensely popular in its contracted modern form, **Tiffany,** but almost unheard of in this full version.

    Theofania, Theophanie

Theophila *Gk.* "God-loving."

    Teofila, Theofila

Theresa *Gk.* "Harvest." May also stem from a Greek place name. The name owes its popularity to two important Catholic saints: the astringent, intellectual mystic St.Teresa of Avila, and the humble young nun, St.Thérèse of Lisieux. It seems to have spread from Catholic families to wider acceptance and was especially common in the 1960s.

    Teresa, Teresina, Terezinha, Teri, Terry, Tessa, Thérèse, Theresina, Theresita, Tracey, Treesa

Thomasina *(Fem.* **Thomas)** *Heb.* "Twin." **Thomasin** was the earliest form, replaced by Thomasina in the Victorian era, and **Tamsin** a hundred years later. Now quite scarce.

    Tamsin, Thomasine

Thora *Scan.* "Thor's struggle." Thor is the Norse god of thunder.

    Thyra, Tyra

Tia *Sp.* "Aunt." Probably used as a first name with little reference to its actual meaning but fondness for its sound.

    Thia, Tiana, Tiara

Tiffany *Gk.* "God's appearance." Literally, **Theophania.** Traditionally used for babies born on Epiphany, the day when the Three Kings first saw the Christ Child. Now associated with Tiffany & Co., the New York City jeweler. The name has become shorthand for upper-class luxury and was hugely popular in the 1980s. By 1990, it was sliding down the list of popularity.

Theophanie, Tiffani, Tiffeny, Tyffany

Tina Diminutive of **Christina** and so on. Used in the 20th century but especially popular in the 1960s.

Teena, Tena, Tine, Tiny

Tita Probably derived from Spanish diminutives such as **Martita**; may be considered a feminization of **Titus** (or **Tito**).

Teeta, Tyta

Titania *Gk.* "Giant." The Titans in Greek mythology were a race of giants. A more familiar use of the name, though, is the Queen of the Fairies in Shakespeare's *A Midsummer Night's Dream.* Easily confused with the more familiar **Tatiana.**

Tania, Tita, Titaniya, Titanya, Tiziana

Toni Diminutive of **Antoinette** (*Lat.* "Beyond price, invaluable").

Toinette, Toney, Tonia, Tonie, Tonina

Topaz *Lat.* Jewel name. Less common than **Ruby** or **Pearl,** but a good candidate for a November baby (it is that month's birthstone) or for a baby with topaz (golden) coloring.

Tori Diminutive of **Victoria** (*Lat.* "Victory").
> **Torey, Toria, Torie, Torrey**

Toya Modern name in the United States, perhaps a diminutive of **Latoya,** one of the most popular "La-" names. It has no particular meaning.
> **Toia**

Tracy Diminutive of **Theresa** (*Gk.* "Harvest"). First used in numbers in the 1940s, probably in response to the film *The Philadelphia Story,* whose main character is named Tracy Lord. This touched off a long period of popularity that is now distinctly fading.
> **Tracee, Tracey, Traci, Tracie**

Tricia Diminutive of **Patricia** (*Lat.* "Aristocratic").
> **Trish, Trisha**

Trina Diminutive of **Katrina** (*Gk.* "Pure").
> **Treena, Treina, Trine, Trinette**

Trixie Diminutive of **Beatrice** (*Lat.* "Bringer of gladness").
> **Trix, Trixee, Trixy**

Twyla Modern name of uncertain meaning and derivation.
> **Tuwyla, Twila, Twilla**

Uma *Sanskrit.* "Flax or turmeric." Uma is also the name of the Indian goddess Sakti, in her guise as light, and is a Hebrew name meaning "nation."

    Ooma

Una *Lat.* "One." The origin of the name may be Irish, though its Celtic meaning is lost. Very unusual.

    Oona, Oonagh

Undine *Lat.* "Little wave." In mythology, Undine is the spirit of the waters. Edith Wharton created a character in *The Custom of the Country* who was named Undine for the hair-curling (or "waving") tonic that had made her father rich.

    Ondina, Ondine, Undina

Urit *Heb.* "Brightness."

    Urena, Uriya, Urith

Ursula *Lat.* "Little female bear." Saint Ursula was a much-venerated virgin martyr, allegedly executed by Attila the Hun, though her story has little basis in fact. The name was most popular in the 17th century. Fans of Disney cartoons will be bound to associate it with the overweight octopus sea-witch in *The Little Mermaid*.

    Orsa, Orsala, Orsola, Ulla, Ursa, Ursala, Ursule, Ursuline

Uta Origin unclear. Possibly diminutive of **Otthild** (*OG.*
"Prospers in battle").

> **Utte, Yuta**

Val Diminutive of **Valentina** and **Valerie**. Occasionally an
independent name.

Valentina *Lat.* "Strong." This name and **Valerie** come from
the same Latin root. **Valentia** was the earliest form, but it
entered the modern age as Valentina. **Valentine** is used
for both boys and girls, and the early Christian martyr for
whom the holiday is named was male.

> **Tina, Val, Valentia, Valentine, Valenzia**

Valerie *Lat.* "Strong." The French form of an early Christian
name (**Valeria**) that was revived at the turn of the 20th
century. It was very popular in the middle of the 20th
century, less so now.

> **Val, Valaria, Valarie, Valeria, Valeriana, Valery**

Vanessa Literary name invented by *Gulliver's Travels* author
Jonathan Swift. Suddenly leaped into everyday use in the
middle years of the 20th century, achieving some popularity in the 1970s and quite considerable use recently.

> **Nessa, Vanesse, Vannessa, Vania**

Velma Origin disputed. Possibly diminutive of **Wilhelmina**
(*OG.* "Will-helmet"), possibly a late 19th-century invention.
In general use since the 1920s but not fashionable.
> **Vehlma, Vellma**

Venetia Place name. Never reached the stature of that other
great Italian tourist mecca, **Florence.** Cropped up from
the 17th century onward; use increased in the 19th century, but the name would still be considered a bit fanciful.
The English form, **Venice,** is also used occasionally.
> **Vanecia, Venezia, Venise**

Venus Name of the Roman goddess of love and beauty.
Used in Britain in the 16th century through the 19th, but
it is very scarce now. It creates a lot of expectations for a
female baby.
> **Venusa, Venusita**

Vera *Slavic.* "Faith"; *Lat.* "Truth." Use by two popular novelists
in the late 19th century promoted the name to high fashion, but it is hardly found now.
> **Veira, Verena, Verushka**

Verbena *Lat.* "Holy plants." Originally referred to olive, laurel,
and myrtle, plants with spiritual significance to the Romans.
In modern times, a class of plants with medicinal properties
and, frequently, pleasant scents.

Verena *Lat.* "True." Derives from the same root as **Vera.**
Primarily English use.
> **Varena, Varina, Veryna**

Verity *Lat.* "Truth." Puritan virtue name, much less common
than **Constance, Hope, Prudence,** and so forth.
Veretie, Veritie

Verna *Lat.* "Springtime." Use spans the late years of the 19th
century to the middle of the 20th century, but the name
has a dated air and is rare today.
Verda, Verne, Verneta

Verona Diminutive of **Veronica.** Also the name of a northern
Italian city well known to tourists, so it may be used by
reminiscent parents.
Varona

Veronica *Lat.* "True image." Or variant of **Bernice** (*Gk.* "She
who brings victory"). According to a legend that sprang
up in the Middle Ages, a young girl wiped Jesus's sweat-
ing brow on his way to Calvary. The handkerchief she
used later showed a perfect image of his face. (Three
separate Italian churches now claim to own this holy
relic.) The name first appeared in Britain in the 17th century, spread beyond Catholic families in the 19th century,
and became popular in the 1950s.
Ronna, Ronnie, Ronny, Veranique, Vernice,
Veronice, Veronicka, Veronika, Veroniqua,
Véronique

Vesta *Lat.* The Roman household goddess. Her altar was
tended by six virgins (the "vestal virgins") who were kept

under severe discipline. They were buried alive if they lost
their virginity. Most common in the late 19th to early 20th
century.

Victoria (*Fem.* **Victor**) *Lat.* "Victory." Extremely common in
Christian Rome but curiously not fashionable during the
reign (1837–1901) of the woman who gave her name to
the Victorian age. Most recently popular in the 1950s and
1960s, but daughters in those days were probably called
Vicky. Parents who use it now are more likely to insist on
the whole mouthful, or **Tori** in a pinch. Victoria hovered in
the top 20 American girls' names from 1993 to 2000, but
use has slowed a bit.

> Tori, Toria, Tory, Vickey, Vicki, Vicky, Victoriana,
> Victorie, Victorina, Victorine, Victory, Viktoria,
> Viktorina, Viktorine, Vittoria

Violet *Lat.* "Purple." A flower name in longer use than most.
Occurred first in the 1830s and lasted nearly a hundred
years, but it has always been more popular in Britain
(whose cool, damp climate is more hospitable to the spring
flowers). **Viola** has been a less-used choice.

> Iolande, Iolanthe, Jolanda, Jolanta, Vi, Viola,
> Violaine, Violanta, Violante, Violetta, Violette,
> Yolanda, Yolantha, Yolanthe

Virginia *Lat.* "Virgin." The name probably derives from a
Roman clan name, but the current meaning has been as-

sumed for hundreds of years. A great favorite in the United
States from the mid-19th century to the mid-20th; the first
child born in the United States with this name was Virginia
Dare in 1597. The state of Virginia was named in compliment to the Virgin Queen, Elizabeth I. A good candidate for
21st-century revival.

> **Geena, Genya, Gigi, Gina, Ginella, Ginger, Ginia,
> Ginnie, Ginny, Ginya, Jinnie, Jinny, Virgie,
> Virgine, Virginie**

Vita *Lat.* "Life." Also occasionally a nickname for **Victoria.**

Viva *Lat.* "Alive." Most familiar from the expression meaning
"Long live…" as in *"Viva l'Espana"* or *"Vive la France."*

> **Viveca, Vivva**

Viveca *Scan.* "Alive." Variation of **Viva.**

> **Viveka, Vivica**

Vivian *Lat.* "Full of life." Used for boys in Britain (although
infrequently), generally for girls in the United States. In
spite of the early martyr Saint Vivian, the name has been
current only since the 19th century and has never been a
real favorite.

> **Bibi, Bibiana, Bibiane, Bibyana, Vibiana, Viv, Vivi,
> Viviana, Viviane, Vivie, Vivien, Vivienne, Vivyan**

Wanda Probably a Slavic tribal name, though some sources suggest *OG.* "Wanderer." Use has been pretty well confined to the middle of the 20th century.

    Vanda, Wahnda, Wannda, Wenda, Wonda

Wendy Literary name coined by James Barrie for the human heroine of *Peter Pan*. The parents who used it in great numbers in the middle of the 20th century may have been inspired by either the musical play or the animated movie. Some, wishing to call a daughter Wendy, no doubt named her **Gwendolyn,** but the names aren't actually related.

    Wenda, Wendaline, Wendi, Wendie

Whitney *OE.* Place name: "white island." Boy's name that became hugely popular for girls in the early 1980s, possibly because of its connotations of old wealth. It was sliding out of the top 100 names by the early 1990s and is now almost an oddity.

    Whitnee, Whitny

Wilhelmina *OG.* "Will-helmet." Despite the number of variants spawned by the name, it hasn't been very popular in any form. Probably used more often to honor a beloved relative named **William** rather than on its own merits.

Billa, Billee, Billie, Billy, Elma, Guglielma, Guillemine, Helma, Mina, Minna, Minnie, Vilma, Wilhelmine, Willa, Willeen, Wilma, Wilmot

Winifred *Welsh.* "Holy peacemaking." Also often explained as Old German for "friend of peace." Popular in Britain for fifty years around the turn of the 20th century but infrequently used otherwise.

Fred, Freddy, Winefride, Winifryd, Winnie

Winola *OG.* "Charming friend."

Winona *Sioux Indian.* "Firstborn daughter."

Wenona, Wenonah, Wynnona

Wren *OE.* Bird name: A wren is a small brown songbird.

Wynne *Welsh.* "Fair, pure." Uncommon, simple, but distinctive in a way that may appeal to today's parents.

Winne, Winnie, Wynn

Xanthe *Gk.* "Yellow." A description of someone's coloring. Almost unknown.

Xantha, Xanthia, Zanthe

Xaviera (*Fem.* **Xavier**) *Basque.* "New house." Given some exposure by Xaviera Hollander, the author of a book that caused some stir in the early 1970s. It was called *The Happy Hooker.*

> Exaviera, Zaveeyera, Zaviera

Xenia *Gk.* "Welcoming." Occurs once in a while as **Zenia.**

> Xeenia, Xena, Zena, Zenia, Zina, Zyna

Yaffa *Heb.* "Lovely."

> Jaffa, Yaffah

Yaminah *Arab.* "Suitable, proper."

> Yamina, Yemina

Yasmin *Arab.* "Jasmine." A variation of a flower name that was quite popular in the late eighties and early nineties.

> Yasmeen, Yasmena, Yasmine

Ynez *Sp.* Variation of **Agnes** *(Gk.* "Pure").

> Ines, Inez, Ynes, Ynesita

Yoko *Jap.* "Good, positive." Would probably be unknown outside Japanese families without the fame of Beatle wife Yoko Ono.

Yolanda *Gk.* "Violet flower." The Spanish version of **Violet.** Used in English-speaking countries in the 20th century, particularly during the 1960s.

Iolande, Iolantha, Iolanthe, Jolan, Jolanne, Jolanta, Yolande, Yolantha

Yonina *Heb.* "Dove."

Yona, Yonit

Ysanne Modern name that is a combination of **Ysabel** and **Anne.** Found in Britain.

Ysande, Ysanna

Yudit *Heb.* "Praise."

Judit, Yehudit, Yudita, Yuta

Yvonne (*Fem.* **Ivo**) *Fr.* from *OG.* "Yew wood." Since yew wood was used for bows, Ivo may have been an occupational name meaning "archer." The most common male form is probably **Yves,** but Yvonne is more widespread in English-speaking countries. It was particularly popular in Britain in the 1970s.

Evonne, Ivonne, Yvetta, Yvette

Zada *Arab.* "Fortunate, prosperous."

Zadie, Zaida, Zayeeda

Zahira *Arab.* "Brilliant, shining."

Zaheera, Zahirah

Zahra *Arab.* "White" or "flower."

    Zahrah

Zandra Variant of **Sandra**; diminutive of **Alexandra** (*Gk.* "Defender of mankind").

    Zahndra, Zohndra, Zondra

Zanna Diminutive of **Susanna** (*Heb.* "Lily").

    Zana, Zannie

Zara *Heb.* "Eastern brightness, dawn." May also be a form of **Sarah** (*Heb.* "Princess"). Literary name used often over the centuries for exotic characters.

    Zarah, Zarina

Zelda Diminutive of **Griselda** (*OG.* "Gray fighting maid"). The original name has long been eclipsed by this nickname, which was made famous by F. Scott Fitzgerald's glamorous but unstable wife.

    Selda, Zelde, Zellda

Zena Variation of **Xenia** (*Gk.* "Welcoming"). This is the slightly more common form of the name.

    Zeena, Zenia, Zina

Zita *Gk.* "Seeker." Also diminutive of **Rosita, Teresita,** and so on. The name of the last Hapsburg empress, who was given the name at the turn of the 20th century when it was at its most popular.

    Zeeta, Zyta

Ziva *Heb.* "Brilliance, brightness."

    Zeeva, Ziv

Zizi *Hung.* Diminutive of **Elizabeth** (*Heb.* "Pledged to God").
Analogous to **Zsa Zsa,** the Hungarian diminutive of
Susan.
    Zsi Zsi

Zoe *Gk.* "Life." Currently popular in Greece and catching on
strongly in English-speaking countries, especially Britain.
    Zoeline, Zoelle, Zoie, Zoila, Zoya

Zola *It.* "Lump of earth." Probably used more for its sound
than for its meaning.
    Zoela

Zora *Slavic.* "Dawn's light."
    Zorah, Zorina, Zorya

Zsa Zsa *Hung.* Diminutive of **Susan** (*Heb.* "Lily"). Made
famous by actress and celebrity Zsa Zsa Gabor.
    Zsuzsa, Zsuzsann

Aaron *Heb.* "Exalted, on high." In the Old Testament, Aaron was the brother of Moses. The name was unusual until the 17th century, when so many Old Testament names first came into prominence. It has been widely used, especially in the United States, since the 1970s.

    Aarron, Aharon, Arand, Arin, Aron, Arron

Abbott *Heb.* "Father." An abbot is the head of a monastic community, so the original bearers of this name (as a surname) may have worked for an abbot. Its use as a first name occurred mostly in the 19th century.

    Ab, Abbot, Abott

Abdul *Arab.* "Servant of." Often used in combination with another name, as in "Abdullah" or "servant of Allah."

    Ab, Abdal, Abdel, Abdoul, Abdullah

Abe Diminutive of **Abraham**. *Heb.* "Father of many."

> **Abey, Abie**

Abel *Heb.* "Breath." Abel was the younger son of Adam and Eve who was slain by his older brother, Cain. Abel has survived with steady use ever since the 6th century, and surprisingly enough, **Cain** also occurs from time to time.

> **Abe, Abell**

Abir *Heb.* "Strong."

> **Abeer, Abeeri, Abiri**

Abisha *Heb.* "Gift of God."

> **Abidja, Abidjah, Abijah, Abishai**

Abner *Heb.* "My father is light." Old Testament name that came to some prominence in the late 16th century.

> **Ab, Abby, Abna, Avner**

Abraham *Heb.* "Father of many." First of the Hebrew patriarchs. In the Bible, Abraham has a son named Isaac when he is 100 and his wife, Sarah, is 90. The name was popular while Abraham Lincoln was president (even more so after his assassination) but has faded from use since 1900.

> **Abarran, Abe, Abrahamo, Abrahan, Abram, Avram, Avrom, Bram, Ibrahim**

Absalom *Heb.* "Father is peace." The handsome son of King David who connived to steal his father's throne. He died in battle, and his father lamented, "Would God I had died for thee, O Absalom, my son, my son!"

> **Absalon, Abshalom, Absolon**

Ace *Lat.* "Unity." Connotations of superiority come from the fact that the ace is the playing card with highest face value.

Acer, Acey, Acie

Achilles *Gk.* Place name; also hero of the *Iliad*, as the greatest of the Greek heroes fighting the Trojans. He was all but invulnerable, having been dipped in the River Styx by his mother. She held him, however, by the heel, which was thus his one weak point; hence "Achilles' heel."

Achill, Achille, Achillea, Achilleas, Akil, Aquilles, Quilo

Achim *Heb.* "God will judge."

Acim, Ahim

Adam *Heb.* "Son of the red earth." In the Bible, God created Adam—the first man—out of the "red earth" and breathed life into him. An appropriate name for the first boy in a family that has produced many girls.

Ad, Adamo, Adams, Adan, Addams, Adem

Adar *Heb.* "Noble."

Adel *OG.* "Noble, highborn." More familiar as a particle of other names.

Adal, Edel

Adham *Arab.* "Black."

Adolph *OG.* "Noble wolf." The Latinized form **Adolphus** arrived in Britain in the mid-19th century, having been a German and Swedish royal name and also a saint's name.

Almost unheard of since the rise of Adolf Hitler and World War II.

Ad, Addolf, Adolf, Adolfo, Adolphe

Adonis *Gk.* In Greek mythology, Adonis was a young man so beautiful that Aphrodite, goddess of love, became enamored of him. The name has come to epitomize male beauty.

Addonis, Adohnes, Adones

Adrian *Lat.* "From Adria"—a northern Italian city. First popular in the 1950s in Britain and used also as a woman's name, though it seems to be holding steady as a choice for male children.

Adriano, Adrien, Adrino, Aydrian, Aydrien, Hadrian, Hadriano, Hadrien

Aeneas *Gk.* "He who is praised." The Trojan hero of Virgil's *Aeneid*. Legend has it that he founded the Italian colony that was the origin of Rome.

Aineas, Eneas, Enné, Enneas

Ahab *Heb.* "Father's brother." A pleasant way to honor an uncle, though literary types may be reminded of the mad sea captain in Herman Melville's novel *Moby Dick*.

Ahmed *Arab.* "Greatly praised." Name often used for the prophet Muhammad and favored by Muslims in the United States. The name is in fact commonly used throughout the Islamic world.

Achmad, Achmed, Ahmaad, Ahmad, Amed

Aidan *Gael.* "Fire." Saint Aidan was a 7th-century Irish monk. The name is also used for girls.

> Aidano, Aiden, Eidan, Eiden

Aimery *Teut.* "Hardworking ruler."

> Aimerey, Aimeric, Aymeric, Imre

Akbar *Arab.* "Great."

Akim *Rus.* Diminutive of **Joachim**. *Heb.* "God will judge."

Akmal *Arab.* "Perfect."

> Aqmal

Alan *Ir. Gael.* Possible meanings: "rock" or "comely." Widely used in the Middle Ages, then again from the 19th century to the late 20th, with a boom around the 1950s influenced by the popularity of actor Alan Ladd. Now waning like most fifties names.

> Al, Alain, Alann, Alano, Alin, Allan, Allen, Alleyn, Alleyne, Allie, Allin, Allyn, Alun

Alastair *Scot. Gael.* Variation of **Alexander** (*Gk.* "Man's defender"). Generally a Scottish name, though it appears occasionally throughout the English-speaking world. Most of the variants are different phonetic spellings of the name.

> Al, Alaistair, Alasdair, Aleister, Alistair, Alystair, Alyster

Albert *OE.* "Highborn, brilliant." Most widely used during the lifetime of Queen Victoria's German prince consort, Albert. Her many children and grandchildren carried the name to most of the royal families in Europe, but her eldest son's first move as king was to drop it. Out of style since the 1920s.

> Adalbert, Adalbrecht, Ailbert, Al, Alberto, Albrecht, Aubert, Bert, Bertie, Berty, Delbert, Elbert

Alden *OE.* "Old friend." Surname transferred to first name, but it is unusual.

> Al, Aldin, Aldwyn, Eldin

Aldo *OG.* "Old." An Italian name that is occasionally used in the United States.

> Aldus, Alldo

Alem *Arab.* "Wise man."

> Alerio

Alexander *Gk.* "Man's defender." Given great prominence by Alexander the Great and steadily used worldwide, as the numerous variants show. Hovering in or just below the top 20 American boys' names since 1999, Alexander seems to be getting more popular without being trendy.

> Al, Alasdair, Alastair, Alcander, Alec, Aleck, Aleco, Alejandro, Alejo, Alek, Aleksander, Aleksandr, Alessandre, Alessandro, Alex, Alexandre, Alexandros, Alexei, Alexis, Alick, Alister, Iskander, Sacha, Sander, Sandor, Sandro, Sandros, Sandy, Sascha, Sasha, Saunder, Sikander, Xander, Zander, Zandro, Zandros

Alexis *Gk.* "Helper." Usually thought of as a diminutive of **Alexander,** though it has a different etymological root. More commonly a girl's name.

> **Aleksei, Aleksi, Aleksios, Alexei, Alexey, Alexi, Alexios**

Alfred *OE.* "Counsel from the elves." After wide medieval use, the name fell out of sight until a 19th-century revival; Queen Victoria even named her second son Alfred. Out of fashion since the 1920s.

> **Ailfrid, Al, Alf, Alfie, Alfredo**

Algernon *OF.* "Wearing a mustache." A first name in several hugely powerful English aristocratic families. The name was given wider use in the latter half of the 19th century in Britain. Oscar Wilde used it for a brainless fop in *The Importance of Being Earnest.*

> **Algernone, Algy, Allgernon**

Ali *Arab.* "The high, exalted one."

> **Aly**

Alonzo Variation of **Alphonse** (*OG.* "Ready for battle").

> **Alanso, Allonzo, Alonso**

Aloysius *OG.* "Famous fighter." Latinized version of **Luigi** or **Louis,** also related to **Clovis** and **Ludwig.**

> **Alois, Aloisius, Lewis, Ludwig**

Alphonse *OG.* "Ready for battle." **Alfonso** is a royal name in Spain and thus very popular there.

> **Affonso, Alfonso, Alfonzo, Alonso, Alonzo, Alphonso**

Alvin *OE.* Several possible sources: the second element, "vin," means "friend"; "Al-" could indicate "elf," "noble," or "old."

> **Ailwyn, Al, Alvan, Alwin, Alwyn, Aylwin, Elvin, Elwin, Elwyn**

Amadeo *Sp.* from *Lat.* "Loved by God." The Latin version is Amadeus, given great prominence by the 1984 film about Mozart.

> **Amadeus, Amado, Amédé, Amyas, Amyot**

Amasa *Heb.* "Bearing a burden." Occasionally used in the 19th century but little known today.

Ambrose *Gk.* "Ever-living." Saint Ambrose was the 4th-century bishop of Milan who baptized Saint Augustine.

> **Ambroeus, Ambrogio, Ambroise, Ambros, Ambrosio**

Amory *OG.* "Home ruler." Variation of **Emery.** F. Scott Fitzgerald used this name for Amory Blaine, the hero of his first best-selling novel, *This Side of Paradise.*

> **Aimory, Amery**

Amos *Heb.* "Borne, carried." A prophet of the Old Testament. The name was infrequently used in the 20th century.

Anastasius *Gk.* "Resurrection." Much more common in the feminine version, **Anastasia.**

> **Anastas, Anastasio, Anasto**

Anatole *Gk.* "From the east." Anatolia is a region of Turkey, which, of course, is east of Greece.

> **Anatoly, Antal**

Anders *Scan.* Variation of **Andrew.**
> Ander, Andersson

André *Fr.* Variant of **Andrew.** Traditionally parents have chosen English-style names for boys in the United States, but
this preference seems to be changing, and names with a
foreign flair are inching into acceptability if not trendiness.
> Andras, Andrei, Andres, Andrey

Andrew *Gk.* "Masculine." In the Bible, Andrew was the first
of the twelve apostles. Legend has it that after his crucifixion on an X-shaped cross, his bones were transported
to Scotland, where he is patron saint. This is a perennial
favorite, in the top 10 of boys' names in the United States
since 1980.
> Aindreas, Anders, André, Andrea, Andreas,
> Andrej, Andres, Andrewes, Andrews, Andrey,
> Andro, Andros, Andy, Drew

Angel *Gk.* "Messenger." **Angelo** is most often used now,
even in English-speaking countries, as Angel is usually
considered a girl's name (although in Thomas Hardy's
1891 novel *Tess of the D'Urbervilles,* a major character is
named Angel Clare).
> Angell, Angelo, Anjelo

Angus *Scot. Gael.* "Sole or only choice." In Celtic mythology
Angus Og is a god of such attractive traits as humor and
wisdom.
> Anngus, Ennis, Gus

Anselm *OG.* "God-helmet." Saint Anselm was archbishop of
Canterbury in the 12th century and one of the formative
influences on medieval Christian thought.

> **Ansel, Anselmo, Elmo**

Anthony *Lat.* Clan name of the Romans, possibly meaning
"beyond price, invaluable." The 3rd-century hermit Saint
Anthony, who, according to legend, lived alone in the
wilderness for over eighty of his hundred-some years,
is patron saint of the poor. A real standby, in or near the
top 20 since 1975, Anthony seems to be getting more
fashionable.

> **Anntoin, Antoine, Anton, Antonello, Antonino,
> Antonio, Antony, Antuwan, Antwon**

Anwar *Arab.* "Shafts of light."

Apollo *Gk.* "Manly." In classical mythology, Apollo is the god
who drives the sun across the sky in a carriage and also
rules over healing and prophecy, speaking through the
famous oracle at Delphi.

> **Apollon, Apollos, Apolo**

Archer *OF.* "Bowman." Originally a surname indicating oc-
cupation (such as **Baker, Miller,** or **Smith**), mildly popular
in the 19th century.

Archibald *OG.* "Noteworthy and valorous." Brought to Britain
with the Norman Conquest and popular largely in Scotland,
where it was in the top 20 until the 1930s.

> **Archambault, Archer, Archie**

Ariel *Heb.* "Lion of God." In Shakespeare's *The Tempest,* Ariel is a sprite who can disappear at will. The name has the connotation of something otherworldly, and though Shakespeare's Ariel is male, the name is used mostly for girls.

> **Airyel, Ariell, Arik**

Aristotle *Gk.* "Superior." Indelibly associated with the Greek philosopher Aristotle.

> **Ari, Aristotelis**

Armand *Fr.* Variant of **Herman** (*OG.* "Army man").

> **Armando, Armond, Ormond**

Arnold *OG.* "Strength of an eagle." Brought to Britain with the Norman invasion, faded out after the 13th century and briefly revived in the late 19th century.

> **Arnaldo, Arnaud, Arnie, Arnoldo**

Arthur *Celt.* Possibly "bear" or "rock." Linked with King Arthur, the legendary British hero of the Round Table, and often used in the Middle Ages, but unfashionable until the early 19th century, when Arthur Wellesley, the duke of Wellington, vanquished Napoleon.

> **Art, Arthuro, Arturo, Artus, Arty**

Asa *Heb.* "Doctor." Another Old Testament name made popular by the Puritans in the 17th century.

Asher *Heb.* "Felicitous." Old Testament name brought into English use by the Puritans.

> **Ash, Asser**

Ashley *OE.* Place name: "ash tree meadow." Originally a surname that migrated to first-name status, possibly helped along by Ashley Wilkes in Margaret Mitchell's *Gone with the Wind*.

> Ash, Ashleigh, Ashlen

Ashton *OE.* Place name: "ash tree settlement." More popular in the 19th century than now, though this is the kind of name Anglophile parents of the 21st century may make more popular.

> Ashtun, Assheton

Auberon *OG.* "Highborn and bearlike." Also possibly a form of **Aubrey.** Better known as **Oberon,** king of the Fairies in Shakespeare's *A Midsummer Night's Dream*.

> Oberon, Oberron

Aubrey *OF.* "Elf ruler." Originally a man's name that arrived in England with the Norman Conquest.

> Alberic, Aubry, Averey

Augustine *Lat.* Diminutive of **Augustus.** The 5th-century bishop Saint Augustine is famous for the frank *Confessions,* in which he says, "Oh God, make me chaste —but not yet."

> Agostino, Agustin, Augustin, Austen, Austin

Augustus *Lat.* "Worthy of respect." Given historical glamour by Roman emperors and German princely families, who brought it to Britain in the 18th century, when it became very fashionable.

> Augie, Augustin, Austen, Austin, Gus

Austin Oral form of **Augustine,** contracted by everyday speech. Now most often a family name transferred to a first name.

> Austen, Austyn

Avery *OE.* "Elf ruler." Variation of **Alfred** and **Aubrey.**

> Averey

Axel *OG.* "Father of peace"; *Scan.* Variation of **Absalom.**

> Aksel, Axell, Axl

Bailey *OF.* "Bailiff." Occupational name: In the Middle Ages a bailiff was a minor officer of the law.

> Baily, Bayley, Bayly

Baird *Ir. Gael.* "One who sings ballads."

> Bard

Balthasar *Gk.* "God save the king." Along with Caspar and Melchior, one of the Three Kings who brought gifts to the baby Jesus, though they are not named in the Bible.

> Baldassare, Baltasar, Baltazar, Balthazar

Barclay *OE.* Place name: "where birches grow." This is the form most favored in Scotland; **Berkeley** is more common elsewhere.

> Barkley, Barklie, Berkeley, Berkley

Bard *Ir.* Variation of **Baird**.

> Bar, Barde, Bardo, Barr

Barnabas *Heb.* "Son of comfort." In the New Testament, Barnabas is a companion of Paul's and uncle of the gospeler Mark. **Barnaby** is now used more often in Britain.

> Barnabee, Barnabey, Barnabus, Barnaby, Barney, Burnaby

Barnett *OE.* Place name: "from the land that was burned." Or possibly a contraction of the English aristocratic title "baronet." **Baron, Duke,** and **Earl** are other ranks of English nobility used as first names from time to time.

> Barnet, Barney, Barnie, Baronet, Baronett, Barrie, Barron, Barry

Barney Diminutive of **Barnabas**.

> Barny

Baron *OE.* The title of nobility used as a first name.

> Baronicio, Barren, Barron

Barret *OG.* "Bear strength." Used as a first name mostly in the 19th century.

> Barratt, Barrett

Barry *Ir. Gael.* "Sharp, pointed." Also a place name turned into a first name used by both sexes. Possibly influenced by the fame of Sir James Barrie, author of *Peter Pan,* since it cropped up as a first name during the height of his renown. Barry with the "-y" was quite popular in the 1950s in the United States.

>   Barrie

Bartholomew *Heb.* "Farmer's son." One of the twelve apostles. The name was common in the Middle Ages but was not revived in the 19th century as so many medieval names were.

>   Bart, Barthelemy, Barthold, Bartholomaus,
>   Barthlomeo, Barthol, Bartlett, Bartolomeo, Bartow

Bartram *OE.* "Bright raven." *See also* **Bertram**.

>   Barthram

Baruch *Heb.* "Blessed."

>   Baruchi, Boruch

Basil *Gk.* "Royal, kingly." Brought to England by the Crusaders, having been common in the eastern Mediterranean. Unusual in the United States, but more often used in Britain. Also the name of a common herb.

>   Basile, Basileios, Basilic, Basilio, Basilius,
>   Vasilios, Vassily

Bayard *OE.* "Russet-haired." A famous French knight of the 15th century, the Seigneur de Bayard was known as "the irreproachable and fearless."

>   Baiardo, Bajardo, Bay

Beau *Fr.* "Handsome." Diminutive of **Beauregard**. Used somewhat in the United States since the 1970s.

>   Beal, Beale, Bo, Boe

Beauregard *Fr.* "Beautiful gaze." In modern parlance, could also be taken to mean "easy on the eye."

> Beau

Bellamy *OF.* "Handsome friend."

> Bellamey, Bellamie

Ben *Heb.* "Son." Also diminutive of **Benedict, Benjamin, Benson,** and so forth. Now given as an independent name.

> Benn, Benny

Benedict *Lat.* "Blessed." Saint Benedict, founder of a monastic order, brought the name to prominence. **Bennett** is the more common form, especially in the United States, where every schoolchild learns the tale of Revolutionary War traitor Benedict Arnold.

> Ben, Bendick, Benedetto, Benedick, Benedictus, Benedikt, Benicio, Benito, Bennett, Benoit

Benjamin *Heb.* "Son of the right hand." In the Old Testament, the younger son of Jacob and Rachel. Brought into use by the Puritan fondness for Old Testament names and persistent until the end of the 19th century. After several decades of disuse the name came back to great popularity by the 1970s and is now quite standard.

> Ben, Benjamino, Benjey, Benji, Benjiman, Benno, Benny, Benyamin, Benyamino, Binyamin

Bentley *OE.* "Meadow with coarse grass." Place name used as surname, then first name, more common for boys but used occasionally for girls. Irresistibly linked in most minds with the luxurious English cars.

Ben, Bently

Beresford *OE.* Place name: "ford where barley grows." Used as a first name principally at the turn of the 20th century.

Berkeley *OE.* Place name: "where birches grow." In the United States, probably most famous as the San Francisco suburb that is home to a branch of the University of California.

Barclay, Barkley, Barklie, Berk, Berkeley, Berklee, Berkley

Bernard *OG.* "Bear/courageous." Brought to England with the Norman Conquest. Two famous medieval saints bore the name: One was a founder of a monastic order. The other, for whom the shaggy brown and white dogs are named, is patron saint of mountain climbers. A fairly common name until the 18th century, revived a bit around 1920, but now unusual.

Barnard, Barnardo, Barney, Barnhard, Barny, Bern, Bernardo, Bernhard, Bernhardo, Burnard

Bert *OE.* "Shining brightly." Diminutive of **Albert, Egbert, Robert,** and so on. Used more often as a nickname.

Bertie, Burt

Bertram *OG.* "Bright raven." Norman name revived in the Victorian era.

Bart, Bartram, Beltran, Bertran

Bertrand *OG.* "Bright shield." Also possibly a variation of **Bertram**.

Bill Diminutive of **William**. Used occasionally as an independent name.

    Billie, Billy

Blackburn *OE.* Place name: "black brook." Used as a first name mostly in the 19th century. In Scotland, *burn* is still the term for a little brook.

    Blackburne, Blagburn

Blaine *Ir. Gael.* "Slender." Surname used since the 1930s as a first name mostly for boys but occasionally for girls.

    Blane, Blayne

Blair *Scot. Gael.* Place name: "plain" or "flat area." Surname now used as a first name, again more common for boys.

    Blaire

Blake *OE.* Paradoxically, could mean either "pale-skinned" or "dark." Surname used most often in the United States as a first name for either sex.

Blakely *OE.* Place name: "dark meadow" or "pale meadow." *See also* **Blake**.

    Blakelee, Blakeleigh, Blakeley, Blakelie

Bo Diminutive of **Beauregard, Robert,** and **Roberto**. Rare as a given name, more likely to be a nickname.

Boaz *Heb.* "Swiftness." Used for several Old Testament characters (including the second husband of Ruth) and revived with the Puritan passion for Old Testament names.

Boas, Boase

Bob Diminutive of **Robert.** *OE.* "Bright fame." Used independently from time to time. The usual habit for naming, however, is to give the full form of a name, even if the parents never intend to use anything but the nickname.

Bobbie, Bobby

Boone *OF.* "Good." The French adjective is *bon* or *bonne.* Backwoods connotations courtesy of 19th-century explorer Daniel Boone.

Booth *OG.* Place name: "dwelling place." Surname whose 19th-century use as a first name was probably a tribute to Salvation Army founder William Booth. Also made famous in the United States by Lincoln's assassin, John Wilkes Booth.

Boot, Boote, Boothe, Both

Borden *OE.* Place name: "vale of the boar."

Bordin

Boris *Slavic.* "Warrior." Russian playwright Pushkin and composer Mussorgsky both based works on the career of the bloodthirsty 16th-century czar Boris Godunov.

Borris, Borys

Bowen *Welsh.* "Son of the young one."

Bowin

Bowie *Scot. Gael.* "Blond."

Bow, Bowen

Brad *OE.* "Broad." Also diminutive of **Bradley** and other "Brad-" names. Quite scarce as a given name.

    Bradd

Braden *OE.* Place name: "wide valley."

    Bradan, Brayden, Braydon

Bradford *OE.* Place name: "wide river crossing."

Bradley *OE.* Place name: "wide meadow." Used since the mid-19th century more in the United States than in other English-speaking countries.

    Brad, Bradleigh, Bradlie, Bradly

Brady *OE.* Place name: "wide island."

    Bradey, Bradie, Braidy

Bram *Ir. Gael.* "Raven." It is curious that so many names refer to the raven, a bird that historically has stood for death and destruction. Bram, of course, can also be a shortened version of **Abraham.**

    Bramm, Bran, Brann

Brandon *OE.* Place name: "broom-covered hill." Also a variant of **Brendan,** which does not quite share its popularity. Brandon had a surge of trendy popularity in the 1990s but has since subsided.

    Brand, Branden, Brandin, Brandyn

Brendan *Ir. Gael.* "Smelly hair." Very few names actually mean anything as negative as this. The Irish Saint Brendan, known as "the Voyager," is supposed to have sailed as far as the Canary Islands in the sixth century.

Brendin, Brendon, Brendyn, Brennan

Brent *OE.* Place name: "mount, hilltop." Use as a first name dates back only sixty years or so and has been particularly strong in Canada.

Brennt, Brentin, Brenton

Brett *Celt.* "Man from Britain." Publicized by American writer Bret Harte. Quite popular in Australia and steadily used in the United States.

Bret, Brette, Bretton

Brewster *OE.* Occupational name: "Brewer." Transferred to a surname, then to a first name.

Brewer

Brian *Ir. Gael.* Ancient name of obscure meaning, though many sources translate it as "strength." Ireland's most famous king, Brian Boru, liberated the country from the Danes in 1014, and the name has been much favored in Ireland. A spell of popularity in the United States lasted from the 1920s to the 1970s, and though Brian is no longer fashionable, it is still well used.

Brien, Brion, Bryan, Bryant, Bryon

Brock *OE.* "Badger." Unusual transferred surname with mostly American use.

Brockley *OE.* Place name: "meadow of the badger."

Brocklea, Brockly

Broderick *ONorse.* "Brother." Traveled from Ireland to Scotland as a surname.

Broderic, Brodric, Brodrick

Brody *Ir. Gael.* "Ditch."

Brodey, Brodie

Bromley *OE.* Place name: "meadow where broom grows." Broom is a shrub related to heather.

Bromlee

Bronson *OE.* "Brown one's son."

Bron, Bronnson

Broughton *OE.* Place name: "settlement near the fortress."

Bruce *OF.* "From the brushwood thicket." Norman place name brought to fame by the Scottish king Robert Bruce, who won Scotland's independence from England in 1327. Naturally popular as a first name in Scotland and among Americans who cherish Scottish ancestry.

Brucey, Brucie

Bruno *OG.* "Brown-skinned." Saint Bruno was the 11th-century founder of the Carthusian order of monks.

Bruin, Bruino

Bryce Unclear origin; may refer to followers of a 5th-century French bishop, Saint Brice.

Brice

Buck *OE.* "Buck deer." "Buck" was also a 19th-century term for a dandy, or a young man who cut a fine figure. It may have been used first as a nickname.

Bucky

Buckley *OE.* Place name: "meadow of the deer."

Burke *OF.* "From the fortified settlement."

> **Berke, Bourke**

Burnell *OF.* "Small brown one."

> **Burnel, Brunell**

Burton *OE.* Place name: "fortified enclosure." Like many of the older place names, used as a first name in the 19th century.

> **Bert, Burt**

Byron *OE.* Place name: "barn for cows." The term *byre* is still used. Used as a first name probably in tribute to the poet Lord Byron, since it dates from the 1850s.

> **Biron, Byram, Byran**

Caesar *Lat.* Clan name of obscure meaning, possibly "hairy, hirsute." The term *caesarean* or *cesarean* for a surgical delivery of a baby came about because the famous Roman emperor Julius Caesar was born that way. It has become a generic term for emperor, translated into German (*kaiser*) and Russian (*czar*).

> **César, Cesare, Cesaro**

Cal Diminutive of **Calhoun, Calvin,** and so on.

Caleb *Heb.* Either "dog" or "courageous." An Old Testament name brought to America with the Puritans, where it was fairly common until around 1920.

    Cal, Cale, Cayleb, Kaleb, Kayleb, Kaylob

Calvin *Lat.* "Hairless." Roman clan name turned surname. Transferred to first name as a tribute to 16th-century Swiss religious reformer John Calvin, whose thinking deeply influenced the Presbyterian, Methodist, and Huguenot branches of Protestantism. Use in the United States may have been influenced by President Calvin Coolidge.

    Cal, Calvino

Cameron *Scot. Gael.* "Crooked nose." Clan name derived from the facial feature. In Scotland, the Camerons were a powerful clan. Little used as a first name until the middle of the 20th century.

    Cam, Camron, Kameron

Campbell *Scot. Gael.* "Crooked mouth." Name of a very famous Scottish clan, again referring to a distinguishing feature. Use as a first name dates back only to the 1930s.

    Campbel

Carey *Welsh.* Place name: "near the castle." Distinct from **Cary,** which has another source. By the 1950s, this form was usually a girl's name, often a nickname for **Caroline.**

    Carrey

Carl Variation of **Charles** (*OG.* "Man"). Use in the United
  States was fairly steady from 1850 to 1950 (probably as a
  result of intensive German and Scandinavian immigration)
  but dropped off in the 1960s.
  Carel, Karel, Karl

Carleton *OE.* Place name: "farmer's settlement." Only used
  as a first name since around 1880. In the United States,
  usually spelled **Carlton**.
  Carl, Carlton, Charlton

Carmine *Lat.* "Song." Though carmine also means "purplish
  red" (from an Aramaic word meaning "crimson"), the Latin
  source is more likely, since the name is almost exclusively
  used by families of Italian descent.
  Carmen, Carmin, Carmino

Carson *OE.* "Son of the marsh dwellers."

Carter *OE.* Occupational name: "one who drives carts."
  Cartier

Cary *OE.* Place name: "pretty brook." Distinct from **Carey**.
  Use in the 19th century as a first name was quite rare,
  but when actor Archibald Leach renamed himself Cary
  Grant, numerous families suddenly found the name Cary
  appealing.

Casey *Ir. Gael.* "Vigilant." Possibly also a short form of
  Casimir. Made famous by the song about the engineer of
  the *Cannonball Express* train, Casey Jones.
  Cacey, Kasey

Casimir *Slavic.* "Bringing peace." Associated with Poland for her famous 11th-century king, who brought peace to the nation.

 Casimiro, Casmir, Kazimierz, Kazimir

Casper Origin unclear, though many sources suggest Persian: "He who guards the treasure." Originally **Jasper**, Germanicized to **Caspar.** Traditionally one of the Three Kings (perhaps the one carrying the gold) was named Caspar.

 Caspar, Gaspard, Jasper, Kaspar

Cecil *Lat.* "Blind one," from a Roman clan name. Used in Roman times, then resurfaced in the Victorian era, possibly given a boost by the fame of industrialist (and founder of Rhodesia) Cecil Rhodes.

 Cecilio, Cecilius

Cedric *OE.* "War leader." Used in two 19th-century literary landmarks (*Ivanhoe* and *Little Lord Fauntleroy*), which probably increased its popularity in Britain.

 Ced, Cedrick

Chad Origin unclear; possibly *OE.* "Fierce." Saint Chad was a 7th-century English bishop. The name enjoyed a burst of popularity beginning in the late 1960s.

 Chadd, Chaddie

Chaim *Heb.* "Life." Male version of **Eve. Hyman** is more common in English-speaking countries.

 Chayim, Haim, Hayyim, Hy, Hyman

Charles *OG.* "Man." The English term *churl,* meaning "serf,"
comes from the same root. Has been a staple ever since
the era of Emperor Charlemagne and a royal name in
many European countries. In the United States, it was one
of the top 5 names for the first three-quarters of the 20th
century but has since been displaced by other classics
such as **Andrew, Christopher,** and **Nicholas.**

    **Carel, Carl, Carlo, Carlos, Charley, Charlie,
Charlton, Charly, Chas, Chaz, Chip, Chuck, Karl**

Chase *OF.* "Hunter." Quite steadily used.

    Chace, Chayce, Chayse

Chester *Lat.* "Soldier's camp." Place name from Roman
Britain, gradually evolved into a first name most common
in the United States.

    Cheston, Chet

Christian *Gk.* "Anointed, Christian." A girl's name that
(contrary to the usual movement) became a male name,
possibly after the huge success of John Bunyan's *Pilgrim's
Progress* (1684), whose hero is called Christian.

    Chris, Cristian, Kristian

Christopher *Gk.* "Carrier of Christ." The much-loved story of
Saint Christopher is that he lived alone by a river, carrying
travelers across the ford on his back. A child who he was
carrying became almost too heavy to bear and proved
afterward to be the Christ Child. In the modern era, the
name was infrequently used until a revival in the 1940s,

possibly influenced by the popularity of A. A. Milne's *Winnie the Pooh,* whose human hero is called Christopher Robin. Among the top 10 boys' names nationwide.

Chris, Christophe, Christos, Cris, Cristoforo, Kit, Kristofer, Kristos, Topher

Chuck Diminutive of **Charles** (*OG.* "Man").

Clarence *Lat.* "Bright." An alternate source is the title Duke of Clarence created for a 14th-century royal prince. In the late 19th century, prompted by the Victorian interest in the picturesque and medieval, Clarence was immensely popular.

Clarance, Clare, Clarrance

Clark *OF.* Occupational name: "cleric, scholar." Surname transferred to first name, heavily influenced by the fame of actor Clark Gable.

Clarke, Clerc, Clerk

Claude *Lat.* "Lame." Name of a Roman clan that produced the emperor immortalized in Robert Graves's novel (and subsequent TV dramatization) *I, Claudius.* **Claud** was used in the 19th century but not in great numbers.

Claudianus, Claudio, Claudius, Klaudio

Claus Diminutive of **Nicholas** (*Gk.* "People of victory").

Claes, Clause, Klaus

Clay *OE.* Occupational or place name involving clay. Most famous modern bearer was probably Cassius Clay, later Muhammad Ali, the boxing champion; he, in turn, had

originally been named for a 19th-century abolitionist,
American statesman Henry Clay.

Clement *Lat.* "Mild, giving mercy." A name borne by fourteen
popes as well as the author (Clement Clark Moore) of "A
Visit from St. Nicholas."

> Clem, Clemencio, Clemens, Clemente,
> Clementino, Clementius, Klement

Cleveland *OE.* Place name: "hilly area." During the fame of
President Grover Cleveland, several towns were named
after him, and the surname became a first name, though
only in the United States.

> Cleaveland, Cleavon

Clifford *OE.* Place name: "ford near the cliff." Surname transferred to first name, most popular in the late 19th century.

> Cliff, Clyff, Clyfford

Clinton *OE.* Place name: "settlement near the headland."
An illustrious 18th-century governor of New York, De Witt
Clinton, left his name on many New York City locations.
Cannot be used now without reference to former President
Bill Clinton.

> Clint, Klint

Clive *OE.* Place name: "cliff." Given some publicity by a famous English soldier, Robert Clive, for his exploits in India.
Its real popularity in England didn't come until the mid-
20th century. Unusual in the United States.

> Cleve, Clyve

Clyde *Scot.* Place name: The River Clyde penetrates western Scotland as far as Glasgow.

> **Clydell**

Cody *OE.* "Pillow." Some sources suggest "son of Odo." Use as a first name was probably influenced by the fame of Buffalo Bill Cody, frontier scout and entrepreneur, who took his *Wild West Show* around the United States and Europe at the turn of the 20th century.

> **Codey, Codie, Kody**

Cole Diminutive of **Nicholas** (*Gk.* "People of victory").

Colin *Gael.* and *Ir. Gael.* "Young creature." Also diminutive of **Nicholas** (*Gk.* "People of victory"). Well known in the Middle Ages and popular in Britain in the middle of the 20th century, but the name didn't spread in numbers to the United States until quite recently.

> **Collin, Colyn**

Connor *Ir. Gael.* "High longing" or possibly "lover of wolves."

> **Conor**

Conrad *OG.* "Courageous advice." Despite occasional increases in its numbers, a name that has never been widely popular in English-speaking countries.

> **Con, Corrado, Curt, Konrad**

Constantine *Lat.* "Steadfast." The form **Constant** was popular among the Puritans (as a virtue name) and was revived in the 19th century to occasional modern use.

Constantine, the Latin form, was the name of the first Roman emperor, 11 Byzantine emperors, and a royal name in Greece.

Constant, Constantin, Constanz, Costa

Cooper *OE.* Occupational name: "barrel maker."

Corey *Ir. Gael.* Place name: "the hollow." Transferred to a surname and used as a first name for either sex. Also diminutive of "Cor-" names.

Corry, Cory, Currie, Curry

Cornelius *Lat.* "Like a horn." Comes from a famous Latin clan name and was often used under the Roman Empire.

Con, Connie, Cornelious, Cornell, Kornelis, Neil

Corwin *OE.* "Heart's friend or companion."

Corwan, Corwinn, Corwyn, Corwynn

Cosmo *Gk.* "Orderliness, organization." Saint Cosmas, a martyr, was patron saint of the Italian city of Milan, and the name was further spread there by the fame of Cosimo de' Medici, grand duke of Tuscany. His friend the duke of Gordon, took the name to Britain in the 17th century.

Cosimo, Cosme, Kosmo

Craig *Scot.* "Rock." (Think "crag.") Surname that has become a standard first name since its introduction only fifty years ago.

Craigie, Craik, Graig, Kraig

Crawford *OE.* Place name: "ford of the crows." Particularly

well used in Scotland as both a surname and a given
name.

> Crawfurd

Crispin *Lat.* "Curly-haired." Saint Crispin, supposedly a
3rd-century martyr (though there is some doubt about his
legend), is patron of shoemakers, and Henry V fought the
battle of Agincourt on his feast day, October 25. The name
was somewhat popular in Britain in the 17th and 18th
centuries, and was revived in the 1960s, but it has not
spread to the United States in significant numbers.

> Crispian, Crispino, Crispo, Crispus, Crisspin

Crosby *Scan.* Place name: "at the cross."

> Crosbey, Crosbie

Cullen *Ir. Gael.* "Handsome."

> Cullan, Cullin, Cullinan

Curt Diminutive of **Conrad**, **Courtney**, and **Curtis**. Most
common in the United States.

> Kurt

Curtis *OF.* "Polite, courteous." Surname used as a first name,
notably in the United States since the 1950s. Used quite
steadily.

> Curcio, Curt, Curtell, Curtice, Curtiss, Kurtis

Cyril *Gk.* "The lord." Popularity confined to Britain from the
turn of the 20th century to the 1930s.

> Ciril, Cyrill, Kiril, Kyril

Cyrus *Per.* "Sun or throne." Famous Persian emperor who
appears in the Old Testament; he allowed exiled Jews to
rebuild Jerusalem.
> Ciro, Cy

Dale *OE.* Place name: "valley." Originally a surname meaning
"one who lives in the valley." The term *dale* is still used
in parts of England. Most famous as a first name in the
1930s.
> Daile, Daley, Dayle

Dalton *OE.* Place name: "the settlement in the valley."
> Daleton, Dallton

Daly *Ir. Gael.* "Assembly." Common Irish surname used since
the 1940s as a first name.
> Daley, Dawley

Damian *Gk.* Meaning not clear: possibly "to tame," although
the Greek root is also close to the word for "spirit." The
name was revived in various forms (**Damien, Damon**) in
the 1950s, having been neglected since the Middle Ages.
> Daemon, Daimon, Damen, Damiano, Damien,
> Damion, Damon, Damyen

Dana *OE.* "From Denmark." Also possibly a place name referring to an English river. Surname first used as a boy's name in the 19th century but now almost exclusively a girl's name, and a specifically American one.

> **Dane, Danie**

Daniel *Heb.* "God is my judge." In the famous Old Testament story, Daniel is thrown into a den of lions because he insists on praying to his God while a captive in Babylon; he was, of course, rescued by the same God. The name has been used with moderate frequency until a spurt of popularity in the late 1950s, which endures still; the name is one of the top 20 in the United States, England, and Ireland.

> **Dan, Dane, Danek, Daniele, Danilo, Danny**

Dante *Lat.* "Lasting, enduring." Actually a nickname, since Italian poet Dante Alighieri's full name was Durante, and modern use of the name almost always refers to him.

> **Dantae, Dontae, Dontay**

Darius *Gk.* "Rich, kingly." Darius the Great was a renowned emperor of Persia in the 5th century B.C.

> **Darias, Dario, Derry**

Darrel Transferred surname, possibly originated as a French place name such as **Darcy.** There are many forms, of which **Darryl** is the favorite by a nose.

> **Darrell, Darryl, Darryll, Daryl, Derrell**

Darren *Ir. Gael.* "Great." Originally a surname, first used as a
    given name in the 20th century. Its popularity was probably
    influenced by the TV series *Bewitched,* in which the rather
    hapless leading man was named Darren.

> **Darin, Darran, Darryn**

David *Heb.* "Dear one." In the Old Testament, the young
    David used his slingshot to kill the mighty giant Goliath and
    went on to become king of Israel and author of the Psalms.
    He has been a favorite subject of artists, notably sculp-
    tors of the Italian Renaissance such as Michelangelo and
    Donatello. In the United States, the name is used by Jewish
    and Christian families alike, and it was in the top 10 boys'
    names from the 1950s to the early 1990s. Still among the
    top 20 boys' names.

> **Dafydd, Dai, Dave, Davey, Davide, Davies, Davis**

Dawson *OE.* "David's son." Surname that cropped up in the
    Middle Ages.

> **Dawes**

Dean *OE.* Place name: "valley"; or occupational name:
    "church official."

> **Deane, Dino**

Demetrius *Gk.* "Follower of Demeter." It has been infre-
    quently used in English-speaking countries.

> **Dametrius, Demetris, Dimitri, Dmitry**

Dennis *Gk.* "Follower of Dionysius." Dionysos was the classical Greek god of wine, but the name also appears in the New Testament. The name has had alternating centuries of favor and disfavor (16th out, 17th in), reaching the height of its 20th-century popularity around 1920.

Denis, Dennie, Dennison, Denys, Deon, Dionisio, Dionysius

Denzel Cornish place name used as a first name almost exclusively in Britain.

Denzell, Denzil

Derek *OG.* "The people's ruler." Most common of the many anglicized forms of **Theodoric,** popular starting around 1890, peaking in the 1930s.

Darrick, Derick, Derrick, Deryk, Dirk

Dermot *Ir. Gael.* "Free man."

Dermott, Diarmid

Derry *Ir. Gael.* Place name: city in Northern Ireland formerly known as Londonderry. Also short form of **Derek, Dermot,** and so forth.

Derrie

Desmond *Ir. Gael.* "From South Munster." Munster was an ancient kingdom in Ireland. Used in England since 1900.

Des, Desmund

Devon English and American place name. More common for girls than for boys.

Deven, Devin

Dexter *Lat.* "Right-handed"; *OE.* "Woman dyer." Modern use, more common in Britain.
> **Dex**

Dick Diminutive of **Richard** (*OG.* "Dominant ruler").

Didier *Fr.* "Much desired." Male form of **Désirée**; currently popular in France.

Diego *Sp.* Variant of **James** (*Heb.* "He who supplants").
> **Dago**

Dieter *OG.* "Army of the people."

Dietrich German form of **Theodoric** (*OG.* "The people's ruler"). *See also* **Derek**.
> **Dedrick, Deke, Derek**

Dillon *Ir. Gael.* "Loyal." Often confused with its popular homonym, the Welsh **Dylan**.
> **Dillan, Dilon, Dyllon, Dylon**

Dominic *Lat.* "Lord." A name popular among Catholic families, possibly because of the fame of Saint Dominic, founder of an important monastic order. Use has spread since the 1950s. Still more common in Britain than the United States.
> **Dom, Domenic, Domenico, Domingo, Dominick**

Donald *Scot. Gael.* "World mighty." Common in Scotland for centuries and popular elsewhere for some fifty years, peaking in 1925. Less popular since the 1950s, perhaps because Disney preempted the name by giving it to a cartoon duck.

Donal, Donalt, Donnell

Donovan *Ir. Gael.* "Dark." Surname became first name or, in
the case of the pop singer who recorded "Mellow Yellow"
in the late 1960s, only name.

Donavon, Donoven

Dorian *Gk.* Place name: "from Doris," an area in Greece.
Introduced by Oscar Wilde in *The Picture of Dorian Gray;*
the hero of the tale is a beautiful young man who suc-
cumbs to a life of vice. Notwithstanding this discouraging
precedent, the name has had some popularity in the
United States.

Dorien, Dorrian

Douglas *Scot. Gael.* Place name: "black water." The name of
a hugely powerful Scots clan. Its period of great popularity,
which peaked in the 1950s, seems to have been inspired
by the actors Douglas Fairbanks, father and son.

Douglass

Drew *Welsh.* "Wise." Diminutive of **Andrew.** Used as an
independent name since the 1960s.

Dru

Duane *Ir. Gael.* "Swarthy." Used primarily since the 1940s,
predominantly in the United States. **Dwayne** is the most
popular spelling.

Dewayne, Dwayne

Dudley *OE.* Place name: "people's field." Aristocratic family

name in England used as a first name since the 19th
century.

Duke *Lat.* "Leader." Last name transferred to first name,
or possibly a shortened form of the highly unusual
Marmaduke. Current use is probably inspired either by
John Wayne (who was nicknamed "Duke") or the great jazz
musician Duke Ellington.

Duncan *Scot. Gael.* "Brown fighter." A royal name in early
Scotland: There was a King Duncan in 11th-century
Scotland whose cousin Macbeth murdered him.
Shakespeare later picked up the tale in his tragedy
Macbeth.
> **Dunc, Dunn**

Dustin *OG.* "Brave warrior"; *OE.* Place name: "dusty area."
Use of the name, which is quite substantial, is almost certainly influenced by the fame of actor Dustin Hoffman.
> **Dusten, Dusty**

Dwight *Flemish.* "White or blond." Use in the mid-20th
century was probably inspired by President Dwight
Eisenhower.

Dylan *Welsh.* "Son of the sea." Welsh legend tells of a sea
god named Dylan, but modern use of the name, which has
spread well beyond Wales, is probably homage to poet Dylan
Thomas. The best-known example of this tribute is singer
Bob Dylan, whose last name was originally Zimmerman.
> **Dillon, Dyllan**

E

Earl *OE.* "Nobleman, leader." The most popular of the English titles of nobility to be used as a first name, though **Baron** and **Duke** also occur.

    Earle, Erle, Erro

Eden *Heb.* "Pleasure, delight." It is a short step from the Hebrew meaning of the word to its general association with Paradise. The name is used for girls as well as boys.

    Eaden, Edin

Edgar *OE.* "Wealthy spearman." A royal name in Anglo-Saxon England which, like **Edmund**, endured through the Norman invasion and the resulting influx of Norman names. In Shakespeare's *King Lear,* Lear's son is called Edgar. Revived, like many Anglo-Saxon names, at the turn of the 20th century, but the revival was short-lived.

    Eadgar, Edgard, Edgardo

Edmund *OE.* "Wealthy protector." A popular and sainted king of the East Angles in the 9th century gave the name enough popularity to survive the Norman Conquest.

    Eadmund, Eamon, Edmond, Edmondo

Edward *OE.* "Wealthy defender." A name with long-lasting popularity throughout the English-speaking world. Used by kings of England (including Saint Edward the Confessor) since before the Norman Conquest and still a staple in the royal family. Though less of an obvious choice since the 1930s, it is still popular.

> **Eadward, Ed, Eddy, Edouard, Eduard, Eduardo, Edvard, Ned, Ted, Teddie**

Edwin *OE.* "Wealthy friend." Anglo-Saxon name revived at the end of the 19th century and used with some frequency since then.

> **Eadwinn, Edwyn**

Eli *Heb.* "On high." In the Old Testament, Eli was Israel's high priest. This was a very holy name to the Hebrews. The Puritans used it freely, and it persisted through the 19th century but faded after the 1930s.

> **Elie, Ely**

Elijah *Heb.* "The Lord is my God." A great prophet in the Old Testament. Felix Mendelssohn, reputedly Queen Victoria's favorite composer, wrote an oratorio about him in 1846. The name was most popular in the early 19th century.

> **Eli, Elias, Elie, Eliot, Ely**

Elisha *Heb.* "The Lord is my salvation." The successor to Elijah, as recounted in the Old Testament. Puritan name in the 17th century, a bit more widespread in the 19th, and all but obsolete now.

> **Eli, Eliso**

Elliott Anglicization of **Elijah** or **Eli**. Surname first used as a given name in modern Scotland, quite popular in the United States.

Eliot, Eliott, Elliot, Elyot, Elyott

Ellis Anglicization of **Elias.** Surname transferred to first name. Ellis Bell was the pseudonym used by Emily Bronte; when they first began publishing, each of the Bronte sisters chose a name that could be considered masculine.

Ellison, Elliss

Elmer *OE.* "Highborn and renowned." Anglo-Saxon name that has been much more popular in the United States than in Britain, especially in the late 19th century.

Aylmar, Aylmer, Ellmer

Elmore *OE.* Place name: "moor with elm trees."

Elton *OE.* Place name: "old settlement" or "Ella's town."

Alton, Eldon, Ellton

Elvis *Scan.* "All-wise." Variants are rare, since use, as in the case of singer Elvis Costello (né Declan Patrick McManus), is almost always influenced by the fame of Elvis Presley.

Elvio, Elviss

Elwood *OE.* Place name: "old wood."

Ellwood, Woody

Emerson *OG.* "Emery's son." First-name use may be a tribute to Ralph Waldo Emerson, the transcendentalist philosopher and "sage of Concord."

Emil *Lat.* "Eager to please." The French form, **Emile,** took root slightly earlier in English-speaking countries. Used only since the mid-19th century.

Aimil, Emile, Emilio

Emmanuel *Heb.* "God is among us." Used in both the Old and the New Testaments, and as another name for Jesus. Slight use in the 17th century grew gradually right through the 19th, then tailed off. In the United States, **Manuel** is fairly common among Catholics of Hispanic descent, who also use **Jesus** quite freely.

Emanuel, Emanuele, Imanuel, Manny, Manuelo

Emmett Various derivations are possible, including *OG.* "Energetic, powerful"; *OE.* "An ant"; or even a last name relating to **Emma.**

Emmet, Emmit, Emmitt, Emmot, Emmott

Enrico *It.* Variation of **Henry** (*OG.* "Estate ruler"). Use by English-speaking families probably reflects the fame of operatic tenor Enrico Caruso. **Enrique** is the Spanish version of the name.

Enrique, Enzio, Enzo

Ephraim *Heb.* "Fertile, productive." Old Testament name used mostly in the 18th and 19th centuries.

Efraim, Efrem

Erasmus *Gk.* "Loved, desired." The 16th-century Dutch humanist philosopher Geert Geerts wrote as Desiderius Erasmus. (**Desiderius** is the Latin form of Erasmus.) Use of the name was greatest in the latter half of the 19th century.

Erasme, Erasmo

Eric *Scan.* "All-ruler." In spite of the renown of Viking explorer Eric the Red (who colonized Iceland around A.D. 985) and his son Leif Ericsson (who reputedly discovered North America half a millennium before Columbus), Eric was little used until the turn of the 19th century. In the United States top 20 in the mid-1970s.

Arric, Erich, Erik, Eriq

Ernest *OE.* "Sincere." Its great popularity at the turn of the 20th century was only confirmed by Oscar Wilde's play, *The Importance of Being Earnest.* Fell out of use after the 1930s.

Earnest, Ernesto, Ernie, Ernst

Errol Origin unclear, though most sources consider it a variation of **Earl.** The most famous modern Errol was dashing movie actor Errol Flynn.

Erroll, Rollo

Ethan *Heb.* "Firmness, steadfastness." An Old Testament name given fame in the United States by Revolutionary War leader Ethan Allen, who captured Fort Ticonderoga with only 83 men. The name leaped into the top 10 in 2002 after a speedy rise from obscurity.

Aitan, Eitan, Etan, Ethen

Eugene *Gk.* "Wellborn." In use since the early Christian era and chosen by four popes. After centuries of disuse, it was dusted off in the 19th century and became very popular in the United States. No longer in the first rank.

> Efigenio, Eugenio, Evgeny, Gene, Iphigenios

Evan *Welsh.* Variant of **John** (*Heb.* "The Lord is gracious"). Most common in Wales but also quite well used in the United States.

> Euan, Evans, Owen

Everard *OE.* "Boar hardness." Norman name more common as a surname but revived in the 19th century.

> Eberhard, Everardo, Everett, Evrard

Ewan *Scot. Gael.* Unclear origin: perhaps "young man" or a variant of **Eugene** or **Evan.** Use confined to Scotland until the mid-20th century but now spreading.

> Euan, Ewen

Ewing *OE.* "Law friend."

> Ewin, Ewynn

Ezekiel *Heb.* "Strength of God." An important Old Testament prophet. Since the end of the 19th century, very scarce.

> Esequiel, Eziequel, Zeke

Ezra *Heb.* "Helper." Old Testament prophet. The Puritans brought the name to America, where it was most used in the 19th century.

> Azariah, Esra, Ezer

Fairfax *OE.* "Blond."

Faisal *Arab.* "Resolute."
Faysal, Feisal

Falkner *OE.* Occupational name: "falcon trainer."
Falconer, Falconner, Faulkner

Farley *OE.* Place name: "meadow of the sheep" or "meadow of the bulls." Surname transferred occasionally to first name.
Fairlie, Farleigh

Farnham *OE.* Place name: "meadow with ferns." Common surname with a little spurt of late 19th-century use as a first name.
Farnum, Fernham

Farouk *Arab.* "Discerning truth from falsehood."
Faruq, Faruqh

Farquhar *Scot. Gael.* "Very dear one." Mostly Scottish use.
Farquar, Farquarson

Farrell *Ir. Gael.* "Hero, man of courage."
Farrel, Farrill, Farryll, Ferrel, Ferrell, Ferrill, Ferryl

Faust *Lat.* "Fortunate, enjoying good luck." Very rare as a first name, no doubt owing to the literary connotations, for the

legendary Faust sells his soul to the devil. His story was
retold by Marlowe, Goethe, Wagner, and Thomas Mann,
among others.

Faustino, Fausto, Faustus

Fedor *Ger.* Variant of **Theodore** (*Gk.* "Gift from God").

Feodor, Fyodor

Felix *Lat.* "Happy, fortunate." Not common in the United
States, possibly because of a strong association with Felix
the Cat and, more recently, *The Odd Couple*'s Felix Unger.

Felicio, Feliks

Fenton *OE.* Place name: "settlement on the marsh." First
used as a given name in the 19th century but never
widespread.

Ferdinand *OG.* "Bold voyager." A name that has always
been more popular in southern Europe than in the English-
speaking countries.

Ferdinando, Fernand, Hernando

Fergus *Ir. Gael.* "Highest choice." Mostly Scottish use.

Fearghas, Ferguson

Fermin *Sp.* "Strong."

Firmin

Ferris *Ir. Gael.* Possibly derived from **Fergus,** or via **Pierce,**
an Irish variant of **Peter** (*Gk.* "Rock"). The 1986 film *Ferris
Bueller's Day Off* may provide discouraging associations,
though.

Farris, Farrish, Ferriss

Fidel *Lat.* "Faithful." The Puritans named boys Faithful, but Fidel is the modern form.

> **Fedelio, Fidele**

Filmore *OE.* "Very famous." Historically best known under the presidency of Millard Fillmore (1850–1853), but nostalgic rock fans may also remember the famous rock-and-roll venue in San Francisco.

> **Fillmore**

Finlay *Ir. Gael.* "Fair-haired courageous one." Most often used in Scotland, where it is a common last name.

> **Findlay, Findley, Finley**

Finn *Ir. Gael.* "Fair"; *OG.* "From Finland."

> **Fingal, Fionn**

Fitz *OF.* "Son of…" Usually short for one of the "Fitz-" names below. Derives from the Norman *filz* or "son."

Fitzgerald *OF./OG.* "Son of the spear ruler." In the United States, famous as the middle name of John F. Kennedy, and the last name of his grandfather, who was known as "Honey Fitz."

Fitzhugh *OF./OG.* "Son of intelligence."

Fitzpatrick *OF./Lat.* "Son of the nobleman."

Fitzroy *OF.* "Son of the king."

Fletcher *ME.* Occupational name: "arrow maker."

> **Flecher, Fletch**

Floyd *Welsh.* "Gray-haired." Anglicization of **Lloyd.**

Flynn *Ir. Gael.* "Son of the ruddy man."

  Flin, Flinn, Flyn

Folke *Scand.* "People's guardian."

  Folker, Volker, Vollker

Forbes *Scot. Gael.* "Field." Used mostly in Scotland.

Ford *OE.* Place name: "river crossing." Most Americans will automatically associate the name with the car.

  Forden, Fordon

Forest *OF.* Occupational name: "woodsman"; or place name: "woods." Most common in the United States, spelled "Forrest."

  Forester, Forrest, Forrester, Foster

Fowler *OE.* Occupational name: "bird trapper."

Francis *Lat.* "Frenchman" or "free man." France was originally the Kingdom of the Franks. Saint Francis of Assisi gave the name its first fame; though he was named John, he had been nicknamed Francis because his father had him taught French as a boy. The name traveled to England via France, and it was popular in the 17th and 19th centuries. **Frank** is more often used now, probably owing to the rise of the feminine version and homonym, **Frances,** but **Francesco** is the best used form in the United States.

  Chico, Ferenc, Fran, Francesco, Franchot,
  Francisco, Franco, Francois, Frank, Frankie,
  Frans, Franz, Paco, Pancho

Frank Diminutive of **Francis** or **Franklin**. Used as an independent name since the 17th century and very popular at the turn of the 20th century right through the 1930s.

Franc, Franco, Franck

Franklin *ME*. "Free landholder." Surname transferred to first name. Popular in the United States, especially in the 1930s and 1940s as homage to President Franklin Delano Roosevelt. President Franklin Pierce apparently made less of an impression, as his term (1853–1857) did not inspire a surge of infant Franklins.

Francklin, Francklyn

Frazer Derivation unclear, possibly Old English for "curly hair" or an old French place name.

Fraser, Frasier, Frazier

Frederick *OG*. "Peaceful ruler." Taken by the Hanoverian kings to Britain, where it began a steady ascent to great popularity that only faded in the 1930s. No longer fashionable but sufficiently common that it doesn't sound outlandish.

Federico, Federigo, Fred, Frederic, Frederik, Fredric, Friedrich, Fritz

Fuller *OE*. Occupational name: "one who shrinks cloth." The woolen fabric that was such a staple of the medieval English economy needed to be treated by fullers before it was made into clothes. The surname was most often used as a first name in the 19th century.

Fulton *OE.* Place name: "settlement of the fowl" or "people's estate." Surname used as first name: in the United States, possibly a compliment to Robert Fulton, inventor of the steamboat.

Fyodor *Rus.* from *Gk.* "Divine gift." Variant of **Theodore**.
> Fedor, Feodor, Fyodr

Gabriel *Heb.* "Hero of God." Gabriel is an archangel who appears in Christian, Jewish, and Muslim texts. The name was uncommon in English-speaking countries, except for a wave of use in the 18th and 19th centuries, but it is now used quite steadily in the United States, perhaps because of the universality of Gabriel's story.
> Gabe, Gabriele, Gavriel, Gavril

Galen *Gk.* "Healer" or "tranquil." A 2nd-century Greek physician named Galen was for centuries the only authority on the emergent practice of medicine.
> Galin, Gaylen, Gaylin

Gardner *ME.* Occupational name.
> Gardener, Gardiner

Gareth *Welsh.* "Gentle." The name of one of King Arthur's

knights. Used in Britain since the 1930s but rare elsewhere.

> Garith

Garland *OE.* Place name: "land of the spear." *OF.* "Wreath."

> Garlan, Garlen, Garlend, Garlin, Garlind, Garllan

Garrison *ME.* "Protection, stronghold."

Garth *Scan.* Occupational name: "keeper of the garden."
Used as a first name in the 20th century but never widely.

Gary *OE.* "Spear." Popularized by film idol Gary Cooper,
whose name was originally Frank. Very fashionable from
the 1950s to the 1970s and still steadily used.

> Garey, Garrie, Garry

Gavin *Welsh.* "White falcon" or "little falcon." As **Gawain**,
this was the name of one of King Arthur's knights. The
Scottish form, Gavin, has spread from Scotland to broad
acceptance in Britain and is quite widely used in the United
States.

> Gaven, Gavinn, Gavyn

Gene Diminutive of **Eugene** (*Gk.* "Well born"). Used as an
independent name since the late 19th century, especially
in the United States.

> Genio, Geno, Jeno

Geoffrey Variant of **Jeffrey** (*OG.* Meaning unclear, something
to do with "peace"). Norman name popular through the
Middle Ages in Britain and revived in the mid-19th century

after a 350-year rest. The peak of its popularity was the 1970s.

> **Geoff, Geoffery, Geoffry, Jefery, Jeff, Jeffrey**

George *Gk.* "Farmer." The popularity of the dragon-killing Saint George (patron of Boy Scouts, soldiers, and England) is undimmed by the fact that little proof of his existence can be found. George was a royal name in England, and admiration for George Washington in the United States gave the name a parallel popularity in the renegade colonies from the 18th century until the middle of the 20th. Now less common but still a steady presence.

> **Egor, Geordie, Georg, Georges, Georgie, Georgios, Georgy, Giorgio, Giorgios, Gyuri, Igor, Jorge, Jurgen, Ygor**

Gerald *OG.* "Spear ruler." Old name revived in the 19th century. Most popular in the middle of the 20th century but now less common.

> **Geraldo, Gerard, Gerold, Gerrald, Gerrold, Gerry, Girault, Jerrold, Jerry**

Gerard *OE.* "Spear brave." Closely related to **Gerald,** and its use follows a similar pattern. Particularly popular in Ireland.

> **Garrard, Garrett, Gerardo, Gerhard, Gerhardt, Gerrard, Gerry, Girard, Giraud, Jared, Jerarrd**

Gershom *Heb.* "Exile." Old Testament name, appearing, appropriately enough, in Exodus.

> **Gersham, Gershon, Gerson**

Gervase *OG.* Meaning unclear; possibly "with honor." Because of the popularity of Saint Gervase, the name has been steadily used by English Catholics but is otherwise unusual.

> Garvey, Gervais, Gervaise, Gervasio, Gervasius, Jarvey, Jarvis, Jervis

Giacomo *It.* Variation of **Jacob** (*Heb.* "He who supplants").

Gibson *OE.* "Son of Gilbert."

> Gibbes, Gibbons, Gibbs, Gillson

Gideon *Heb.* "Feller of trees" or "mighty warrior." A biblical judge and hero who, with an army of only three hundred men, liberated the Israelites from the Midianites. The latter-day Gideons are the group responsible for placing Bibles in hotel bedrooms.

> Gideone, Gidi, Gidon, Hedeon

Gifford *OE.* Either "brave giver" or "puffy-faced." It is astonishing how rarely the derivations of names mean anything negative; this exception to that rule is used as a first name from time to time.

> Giffard, Gifferd, Gyfford

Gilad *Arab.* "Hump of a camel"; *Heb.* "Monument, site of testimony."

> Giladi, Gilead

Gilbert *OG.* "Shining pledge." Norman name much used in the Middle Ages, but use tapered away to mostly local favor in Scotland and northern England. Very unusual in the United States.

Bert, Gib, Gil, Gilberto, Gill

Giles *Gk.* "Kid, young goat." The link with a shield or shield
bearer (sometimes the translation given for Giles) probably comes from the kidskin of which ancient shields were
made. More widely used in the United Kingdom.

Gilles, Gillis, Gilliss, Gyles

Gillespie *Ir. Gael.* "Son of the bishop's servant."

Gillaspie, Gillis

Gilmore *Ir. Gael.* "Servant of the Virgin Mary."

Gillmore, Gillmour, Gilmour

Gilroy *Ir. Gael.* "Servant of the redhead."

Gilderoy, Gildroy, Gillray, Gillroy

Gino *It.* Diminutive of **Ambrogino** (*Gk.* "Ever-living"),
Luigino, or possibly **Eugene** (*Gk.* "Well born").

Geno, Jeno, Jino

Giovanni *It.* Variation of **John** (*Heb.* "The Lord is gracious").

Gian, Gianni, Giannino, Giovan, Giovanno,
Jovanney

Giulio *It.* Variation of **Julius** (*Lat.* "Youthful").

Giuliano

Giuseppe *It.* Variation of **Joseph** (*Heb.* "The Lord increases").

Glen *Ir. Gael.* Place name: "glen." A glen is a narrow valley
between hills. As a surname, Glen would indicate an ancestor who lived in such a valley.

Glenn, Glennon

Godfrey *OG.* "God-peace." Popular medieval name that faded very gradually to its near disuse today.

> Godfry, Gottfried

Gonzalo *Sp.* "Wolf."

> Gonsalve, Gonzales

Gordon *OE.* Meaning unclear, possibly a place name meaning "hill near meadows" or "triangular hill." Historically associated with Scotland, but principal use has been in the 20th century.

> Gorden, Gordie

Gore *OE.* "Spear" or "wedge-shaped object." *Gore* is also an old term for a small, triangular-shaped piece of land, so this may be considered a place name, denoting an ancestor who lived on or near such a piece of land.

> Goring

Grady *Ir. Gael.* "Renowned." A transferred Irish last name.

> Gradee, Gradey, Graidey, Graidy

Graham *OE.* "Gray homestead." Mostly Scottish name that was popular in Britain in the 1950s without ever being much used in the United States.

> Graeham, Graeme, Grahame

Grant *Fr.* "Tall, big." Another Scottish name, but one that has been more popular in the United States as a first name, probably inspired by President Ulysses S. Grant.

> Grantham, Grantley

Gray *OE.* "Gray-haired."
> Graye, Grey

Grayson *OE.* "Son of the gray-haired man."
> Graydon, Greydon, Greyson

Gregory *Gk.* "Watchful, vigilant." A staple name in the Middle
Ages used by 16 popes and 10 saints. Modern popularity
dates from the 1940s, which means it is probably linked
to actor Gregory Peck's rise to stardom. Like most names
that were very fashionable in the 1950s, it is now a bit out
of style.
> Graig, Greg, Greger, Gregg, Greggory, Gregoire,
> Gregor, Gregorio, Gregorius

Gresham *OE.* Place name: "village surrounded by pasture."

Greville *OF.* Place name used occasionally in Britain.
> Grevill

Griffin *Lat.* "Hooked nose." The name of a mythical beast,
usually half eagle (hence the hooked nose), half lion. Use
as a name may be connected to the frequent heraldic use
of the animal.
> Griff, Griffen, Griffon, Gryffen, Gryffin, Gryphon

Griffith *Welsh.* "Strong chief." Used most often as a first
name in the 16th through 18th centuries. Use is sparing
but increasing.

Gustave *Scan.* "Staff of the gods." A royal name in Sweden,
used elsewhere in Europe in the 17th century, and in

England in the 19th century. American use (which is uncommon) tends to harken back to Scandinavian ancestry.

> Gus, Gustaf, Gustav, Gustavus

Guthrie *Ir. Gael.* Place name: "Windy spot."

> Guthree, Guthrey, Guthry

Guy Unclear origin, though some sources make a case for
French "guide" or Old German "warrior." To Americans, it is
a very English-sounding name.

> Guido

Habib *Arab.* "Loved one."

> Habeeb

Hadden *OE.* Place name: "hill of heather."

> Haddon

Hadley *OE.* Place name: "heather meadow."

> Hadlee, Hadleigh

Hadrian Variation of **Adrian** (*Lat.* "From Adria"). Adria was a
northern Italian city. Roman Emperor Hadrian was responsible for the building of a vast wall across northern Britain,
parts of which still stand.

> Adrian, Adriano, Adrien, Hadrien

Hal Diminutive of **Henry** and **Harold.** In Shakespeare's plays about Henry IV, his son (to become Henry V) is affectionately known as "Prince Hal."

Hale *OE.* Either place name "from the hall," or "healthy hero." Revolutionary War hero Nathan Hale was hanged by the British as a spy. His famous last words on the scaffold were "I regret that I have but one life to lose for my country."

    Hal, Hayle

Halsey *OE.* Place name: "Hal's island."

    Hallsey, Hallsy, Halsy

Halton *OE.* Place name: "estate on the hill."

    Halton, Halten

Ham *Heb.* "Heat." Old Testament name; one of the sons of Noah. Little used; the names of Noah's other sons, Shem and Japheth, are even more rare.

Hamal *Arab.* "Lamb."

    Amahl, Amal, Hamahl

Hamilton *OE.* Place name of several possible meanings such as "home lover's estate" or "hill with grass." It was the surname of several aristocratic British families and made the transition to a first name in the early 19th century.

    Hamelton, Hamil, Hamill

Hamish *Scot.* Variant of **James** (*Heb.* "He who supplants"). Rare outside of Scotland.

Hanford *OE.* Place name: "high ford."

Hank Diminutive of **Henry** (*OE.* "Estate ruler"). Usually a
   nickname rather than a given name.

Hanley *OE.* Place name: "high meadow."
   Handley, Hanleigh, Hanly, Henleigh, Henley

Hans *Scan.* Variation of **John** (*Heb.* "The Lord is gracious").
   Currently very popular in Germany.
   Hannes, Hanns, Hansel

Hanson *Scan.* "Son of Hans."
   Hansen, Hanssen, Hansson

Harding *OE.* "Son of the courageous one."
   Hardinge

Harlan *OE.* Place name: "army land."
   Harland, Harlen, Harlin, Harlyn, Harlynn

Harley *OE.* Place name: "the long field." Familiar to most
   people as half of the name of a great motorcycle, the
   Harley-Davidson.
   Arleigh, Arley, Harlee, Harleigh

Harlow *OE.* Place name: "army hill."
   Arlo, Harlo, Harloe, Harlow

Harmon Variant of **Herman** (*OG.* "Army man").
   Harman, Harmann, Harmonn

Harold *Scan.* "Army ruler." An Anglo-Saxon name revived to
   great popularity in the mid-19th century. It was greatly in
   vogue until the turn of the 20th century but is now rare.
   Hal, Harald, Haroldo, Harry, Herrold

Harper *OE.* "Harp player."

    Harpur

Harrison *OE.* "Son of Harry."

    Harris, Harriss, Harrisson

Harry Diminutive of **Henry** (*OE.* "Home ruler"). Since about 1920, Harry has been used as an independent name about as frequently as **Henry.** In the United States, this may have something to do with admiration for President Harry S. Truman. The cultural reach of Harry Potter may dim this name's utility for a while.

Hartley *OE.* Place name: "stag meadow."

    Hartlea, Hartlee, Hartleigh, Hartly

Harvey *OF.* "Burning for battle" or "strong and ardent." Norman name revived in the 19th century but now uncommon.

    Harvie, Herve, Hervey

Harwood *OE.* Place name: "wood of the hares."

    Harewood

Hashim *Arab.* "Crusher of evil."

    Hasheem, Hisham

Haskel *Heb.* "Intellect."

    Haskell

Hayden *OE.* Place name: "hedged valley."

    Haden, Haydn, Haydon

Hayes *OE.* Place name: "hedged area."

    Hays

Hayward *OE.* Occupational name: "keeper or guardian of the hedged enclosure."

Haywood *OE.* Place name: "hedged forest."

Heywood, Woody

Heath *ME.* Place name: "heath." In Britain *heath* is the name for a large, open space that's not under cultivation.

Hector *Gk.* "Holds fast." One of the great heroes of the Trojan War, though today the verb form "to hector" means to bully or browbeat. Quite steadily used.

Ector, Ettore

Hedley *OE.* Place name: "heathered meadow." Used in Britain in the late 19th century, but rare in the United States.

Headleigh, Headley, Headly, Hedly

Henry *OG.* "Estate ruler." Norman name that took root in Britain and became a royal name of eight kings and, most recently, the younger son of the Prince of Wales. This exposure may give new popularity to a name that was extremely common until the first quarter of the 20th century and is now used less than unusual names such as **Blake**, **Jayden**, and **Wyatt**.

Arrigo, Enrico, Enrique, Enzo, Hal, Hank, Harry, Heinrich, Hendrik, Henri

Herbert *OG.* "Bright army" or "bright warrior." Norman name that faded in the Middle Ages, to be revived enthusiastically in the 19th century. Now unusual.

Bert, Erberto, Hebert, Heriberto

Hercules *Gk.* Meaning not quite clear: possibly "glorious gift" or "glory of Hera." The name of a legendary Greek hero who exhibited incredible strength.

> Ercole, Herakles, Hercule

Herman *OG.* "Army man." Another 19th-century revival of a Norman name, this one especially a favorite in the United States.

> Armand, Ermano, Harman, Harmon, Hermann, Herminio

Hernando *Sp.* Variant of **Ferdinand**. *OG.* "Bold voyager."

Hershel *Heb.* "Deer." As **Herzl**, this name is often used to commemorate Theodor Herzl, an early Zionist.

> Hersch, Herschel, Herschell, Herzel, Herzl, Heschel, Heshel, Hirschl

Hillel *Heb.* "Greatly praised." Sometimes used in honor of the celebrated 1st-century Jewish scholar Rabbi Hillel.

Hilliard *OG.* "Battle guard"; *OE.* Place name: "yard on a hill."

> Hiller, Hillyard, Hillyer

Hilton *OE.* Place name: "hill settlement."

> Hylton

Hiram *Heb.* Meaning not clear, possibly "most noble." Old Testament name infrequently used in the 20th century, though fairly popular in the 19th century.

> Hi, Hirom, Hy, Hyrum

Hobart A particularly American (though unusual) variant of **Hubert** (*OG.* "Bright or shining intellect").

Hobard, Hobert, Hobey, Hobie, Hoebart

Hogan *Ir. Gael.* "Youth."

Holbrook *OE.* Place name: "stream near the hollow."

Brook, Holbrooke

Holcomb *OE.* "Deep valley." *Combe* is a term sometimes used in England for a deep, narrow valley.

Holcombe, Holcoomb

Holden *OE.* Place name: "hollow valley."

Homer *Gk.* "Security, pledge." The name of the classical poet, author of the *Iliad* and the *Odyssey*. More popular in the United States than elsewhere, especially in the 19th century.

Homere, Homero, Homeros, Homerus, Omero

Horace *Lat.* Clan name, possibly meaning "timekeeper." Late 19th-century use may have been inspired in part by the famous Roman poet Horace.

Horacio, Horatio, Horatius, Oratio, Orazio

Horton *OE.* Place name: "gray settlement."

Horten, Orton

Hosea *Heb.* "Salvation." Name of an Old Testament prophet, but less popular, even in the 19th century, than other prophets' names such as **Joel** or **Amos**.

Hoseia, Hoshea, Hosheia

Houghton *OE.* Place name: "settlement on the headland."

Hough

Howard *OE.* Meaning unclear, possibly occupational name indicating a watchman of some kind.

> Howie, Ward

Howell *Welsh.* "Eminent, remarkable."

> Howel, Howells

Howland *OE.* Place name: "land with hills."

> Howlan, Howlen

Hubert *OG.* "Bright or shining intellect." An old European name that was popular around the turn of the 20th century but is now rare.

> Bert, Hobart, Hubbard, Huberto, Hubie

Hudson *OE.* "Hugh's son."

Hugh *OG.* "Mind, intellect." Popular medieval name steadily used (though at a diminishing rate) in the modern era.

> Hughes, Hughie, Hugo

Humphrey *OG.* Meaning unclear but alludes to peace. In the Middle Ages, the form **Humfrey** was used in England, but Humphrey was the usual form from 1700 on. Never immensely popular.

> Humfrey, Humfry, Humphery

Hunter *OE.* Occupational name: "hunter." Used mostly by the Scots.

> Hunt

Hussein *Arab.* "Small, handsome one." A royal name in Jordan.

> Husain, Husayn, Husein

Hutton *OE.* Place name: "settlement on the bluff."
> Hutten

Hyde *OE.* Place name referring to a "hide," a measure of land
in the early Middle Ages. It amounted to about 120 acres.

Hyman Anglicized variant of **Chaim** (*Heb.* "Life").
> Hayim, Hayyim, Hymie, Mannie

I

Ian *Scot.* Variation of **John** (*Heb.* "God is gracious"). One
of the few Scottish names that has achieved really broad
popularity since the beginning of the 21st century.
> Iain, Ion

Ibrahim *Arab.* Variant of **Abraham** (*Heb.* "Father of many").
This form of the name is more common in Muslim countries.

Imad *Arab.* "Support, mainstay."

Immanuel Variant of **Emmanuel** (*Heb.* "God is among us").
> Imannuel, Imanoel, Imanuel

Ingemar *Scan.* "Ing's son." Ing was a powerful god of fertility
and peace in Norse mythology.
> Ingamar, Ingmar

Ingram *OE.* "Raven of Anglia." A first name until the 17th century, now more commonly a surname that is occasionally transferred.

Ingraham, Ingrams

Innis *Scot. Gael.* Place name: "island."

Ennis, Innes, Inness, Inniss

Ira *Heb.* "Watchful." Old Testament name revived in the 19th century but never very popular.

Irving *OE.* "Sea friend." Also a Scottish place name. Used as a first name since the middle of the 19th century.

Earvin, Ervin, Irv, Irvin, Irvine

Irwin *OE.* "Boar friend." Revived from roughly 1860 to the 1940s but infrequently used since then.

Erwin, Irwinn, Irwyn

Isaac *Heb.* "Laughter." In the Old Testament, Abraham's son, born when his father was one hundred years old. The Puritans used the name enthusiastically, and it remained popular through the 18th century, fading very gradually. Very steadily used now, as is **Isaiah.**

Ike, Isaak, Isak, Itzak, Yitzhak, Zack

Isaiah *Heb.* "The Lord helps me" or "salvation of God." Like so many Old Testament names, popular with the Puritans in the 17th century, brought to America, and revived by the Victorians. And now, like **Isaac,** increasingly popular.

Isaias, Isiah, Iziah

Ishmael *Heb.* "The Lord will hear." Old Testament name immortalized in the first line of Herman Melville's *Moby Dick:* "Call me Ishmael."

Ismael, Ismail, Ysmael, Ysmail

Israel *Heb.* Meaning unclear, though some sources suggest "wrestling with the Lord," for this was the name given to Jacob in the Old Testament after his three-day bout with his Lord. Came to be synonymous with the Jewish people and was consequently used as the name for the new Jewish state founded in 1948.

Yisrael

Ivan *Rus.* Variant of **John** (*Heb.* "God is gracious"). Used in English-speaking countries for the last hundred-odd years.

Ifan, Iwan

Ivo *OG.* "Yew wood." Since yew wood was used for bows, the name may have been an occupational one meaning "archer."

Ives, Yves, Yvo

Jack Familiar form of **John** (*Heb.* "The Lord is gracious") or, less often, **Jacob** (*Heb.* "He who supplants"). Currently experiencing quite a little renaissance, possibly because of its slightly rugged, down-home aura.

Jackie, Jacky

Jackson *OE.* "Son of Jack." May indicate an ancestor's admiration for President Andrew Jackson or, in Southern families, Civil War General Stonewall Jackson.

> **Jacksen, Jaxen**

Jacob *Heb.* "He who supplants." In the Old Testament, Jacob, Esau's brother, impersonates his brother at his blind father Isaac's deathbed by covering his hands with a goatskin (since his brother Esau was "an hairy man") to secure blessing meant for the elder son. The most popular boys' name in the United States since 1999.

> **Giacomo, Iakov, Jacobi, Jacoby, Yakov**

Jaden Modern invented name. Something about the ever-popular "J-" sound and the two-syllable cadence has made this name and its variant **Jayden** very fashionable.

> **Jadon, Jayden, Jaydin**

Jamal *Arab.* "Handsome." Very popular in the United States among African-American and Muslim families.

> **Jamel, Jemal**

James English variant of **Jacob** (*Heb.* "He who supplants"). In the New Testament, there are two apostles known as James, though the Old Testament version of the name is always Jacob. The name was popularized by the Stuart kings James I and II, and it has been a stable favorite ever since. Use has diminished a bit since 1990, when it was in the top 10.

> **Diego, Giacomo, Hamish, Iago, Jacques, Jago,**

Jaime, Jamie, Jaymes, Jim, Jimmie, Seamus, Shamus

Jameson *OE.* "Son of James."

Jaimison, Jamieson, Jamison

Jared *Heb.* "He descends." Related to **Jordan**. Old Testament name used by the Puritans. Fairly steady use increased in the 1990s.

Jarod, Jarrard, Jerod

Jarvis Variation of **Gervase** (*OG.* Meaning unclear: possibly "with honor").

Jarvey, Jary, Jervey, Jervis

Jason *Heb.* "The Lord is salvation." The name is actually a variation of **Joshua** formed by biblical translators. Jason was a legendary Greek hero who, after many adventures, recovered the Golden Fleece from an enemy kingdom. The name was in the top 10 from 1971 to 1983.

Jacen, Jay, Jaysen, Jayson

Jasper *Eng.* Variant of **Caspar.** Possibly Persian for "he who guards the treasure." Jasper is also a strikingly colorful variety of quartz.

Gaspar, Jaspar, Jesper

Javier *Sp.* Variant of **Xavier.** Meaning obscure but refers to Saint Francis Xavier.

Havier, Javi, Javiero

Jay *Lat.* "Jaybird." A medieval name that has survived especially in the United States, where it is given to boys and girls alike. Its use may be inspired by the first chief justice of the U.S. Supreme Court, John Jay.

Jefferson *OE.* "Son of Jeffrey." Surname used as a first name. President of the Confederacy Jefferson Davis, who was born in 1808, was probably named for then-President Thomas Jefferson.

> **Jeffers, Jeffersson**

Jeffrey *OG.* Meaning unclear but refers to "peace." Norman name popular through the Middle Ages in Britain and revived in the mid-19th century after a 350-year rest. The peak of its popularity was during the 1970s in the United States, with this form preferred to **Geoffrey.**

> **Geoff, Geoffrey, Jefery, Jeff, Jefferey, Jefferies, Jeffery, Joffrey**

Jeremiah *Heb.* "The Lord exalts." Old Testament prophet who lived in Jerusalem when it fell to the Babylonians. The Book of Jeremiah is so relentlessly gloomy that "jeremiad" has become the term for a lengthy complaint. The Puritans used Jeremiah somewhat, but **Jeremy** has eclipsed it in modern times.

> **Jem, Jeremia, Jeremias**

Jeremy Modern form of **Jeremiah.** One source suggests that the modern penchant for Jeremy was sparked by a 1960s TV series called *Here Come the Brides.* This may be true, since the Jeremy on the show had brothers named **Jason** and **Joshua**—names that were simultaneously fashionable in the late 1970s.

Jem, Jeramey, Jeramie, Jeremie

Jerome *Gk.* "Sacred name." The 5th-century Saint Jerome was responsible for a Latin translation of the Bible. The name was best used in the 16th and 19th centuries.

Gerome, Geronimo, Hieronimos, Jairo, Jeroen

Jesse *Heb.* "The Lord exists." The biblical father of King David.

Jess, Jessie, Yishai

Jesus *Heb.* "The Lord is salvation." Used mostly by families of Latin American origin, but **Joshua,** from the same Hebrew derivation, is tremendously popular across the United States.

Jesous

Jethro *Heb.* "Preeminence." Old Testament name that occurred from time to time until the late 19th century. A flicker of modern use may have been inspired by the rock group Jethro Tull.

Jeth, Jethroe

Jim Diminutive of **James** (*Heb.* "He who supplants"). Used occasionally as an independent name.

Jimi, Jimmy

Joachim *Heb.* "God will judge."

Ioakim, Joaquin, Josquin

Joel *Heb.* "Jehovah is the Lord." Along with **Amos,** the most common of the Old Testament prophets' names, though

Hosea also occurs. Combines two strong recent trends: Old Testament names and those beginning with J.

> Yoel

John *Heb.* "The Lord is gracious." Given a sound foundation by two crucial saints, John the Baptist and John the Evangelist. (There are another thirty-odd significant saints named John.) The name has been used by endless numbers of parents all over the world. In the English-speaking countries, it was the most popular boy's name for over four hundred years. One of the top 10 American names from 1965 to 1985 and in the top 20 since then. The variants below are just a small sampling.

> Euan, Evan, Gianni, Giovanni, Hannes, Hanno, Hansel, Ian, Ioannes, Ivan, Jack, Jan, Jean, Jenkin, Jens, Joannes, Joao, Jock, Johann, Johannes, Johnnie, Johnny, Jon, Jovan, Juan, Juwan, Sean, Shane, Shaun, Shawn, Vanya, Yanni, Zane

Johnson *OE.* "Son of John." Mostly 19th-century use.

> Johnston, Jonson

Jonas *Gk.* Variation of **Jonah** (*Heb.* "Dove"). Jonah is the biblical hero who was swallowed alive by a whale, in whose belly he lived for three days.

> Jonah, Jonaso

Jonathan *Heb.* "Gift of Jehovah." Related to **Nathan** rather than to **John.** In the Old Testament, the great friend of

King David. Used in the 17th century, then neglected from the 18th century until the 1940s. Some of its current extensive use probably comes about because it resembles John.

>Johnathan, Johnathon, Jon, Jonathon

Jordan *Heb.* "Descend." Named after the River Jordan. First used in the Middle Ages by Crusaders returning from the Holy Land. Revived slightly in the 19th century. Popular for both boys and girls, but male use has the edge at the moment.

>Giordano, Jordao, Jordon, Jory, Jourdain

Jorge *Sp.* Variant of **George** (*Gk.* "Farmer").

José *Sp.* Variant of **Joseph.**

Joseph *Heb.* "Jehovah increases." Name that occurs for principal figures in both the Old and the New Testaments of the Bible. It has been slightly less used than **John,** but has nevertheless been a top 20 name in the United States since 1965.

>Giuseppe, Iosef, Iosif, Jessup, Jodie, Joe, Joey, Joop, Joos, José, Josef, Josip, Joss, Joszef, Osip, Pepe, Pino, Sepp, Yusif, Yusuf

Joshua *Heb.* "The Lord is salvation." An Old Testament hero, Moses's successor. Immensely fashionable in the late 1970s and still well used.

>Josh, Joushua, Yehoshua

Josiah *Heb.* "The Lord supports." An Old Testament king of Judah. Most common in the 18th century, now rare.
> Josia, Josias

Juan *Sp.* Variation of **John** (*Heb.* "The Lord is gracious").
> Juwan

Julian *Lat.* Variation of **Julius.** First took hold in the 18th century and became fashionable in the 1950s through the 1970s. Steadily used today.
> Jolyon, Julien, Julyan

Julius *Lat.* Clan name: "youthful." Common in Christian Rome and revived in the 19th century. Now scarce.
> Jule, Jules, Julio

Justin *Lat.* "Fair, righteous." Another name well used by Roman Christians but unusual elsewhere until quite recently. American popularity peaked in 1988.
> Giusto, Justen, Justinius, Justyn

Kaden Modern invented name, analogous to the popular **Jaden** and **Hayden.** Surprisingly well used for a name that was only recently invented.
> Caden, Cayden, Kayden

Kai Modern name, possibly related to *Old Welsh.* "Rejoicing." The Welsh form is spelled **Kay**, which is now considered a woman's name, related to **Katherine.** This version is usually pronounced with a long "-I" rather than a long "-A."

> Kay, Keh

Kalil *Arab.* "Friend."

> Kahlil, Khaleel, Khalil

Kamal *Arab.* "Perfection, perfect."

> Kameel, Kamil

Kareem *Arab.* "Highborn, generous."

> Karam, Karim

Karl *OG.* "Man." Variation of **Charles.** The Germanic form of the name; as **Carl**, it was fairly well used in the United States from 1850 to 1950. "K" spellings are not as readily adopted for boys' names as they are for girls'.

> Carl, Karel, Karol, Karoly

Kedar *Arab.* "Powerful."

> Kadar, Keder

Keenan *Ir. Gael.* "Small and ancient."

> Keenen, Kienan, Kienen

Keith *Scot. Gael.* "Forest." Originally a place name adopted as a first name for non-Scots in the 19th century. Peaked in the 1960s in the United States, but still fairly steadily used.

Kelsey *OE.* Place name, incorporating a word particle that means "island." Has been more frequently used as a girl's name and was very popular in the 1990s.

Kelsie, Kelsy

Kennedy *Ir. Gael.* Some sources suggest "helmet/head,"
while "ugly/head" is also offered, which would make this
one of the rare names to refer to negative characteristics
or habits possessed by ancestors. Use of Kennedy as a
first name may be inspired by President John F. Kennedy.

Canaday, Canady, Kennedey

Kenneth *Ir. Gael.* "Handsome" or "sprung from fire." Originally
a favorite Scottish name that spread starting in the late
19th century. Very popular in the United States in the
1950s and 1960s.

Ken, Kennet, Kennett, Kennith, Kenny

Kent *OE.* Place name: a county in England. Familiar as a
surname and used in the United States as a first name. In
the 1930s and 1940s, monosyllabic names (**Burt, Clark,
Kirk**) seemed to project a manly aura and enjoyed a con-
sequent burst of popularity.

Kennt, Kentt

Kenyon *Ir. Gael.* "Blond."

Kerry Irish place name: Kerry is a county in southwestern
Ireland. Also, according to some sources, "dark-haired."
Used more often for girls.

Kearie, Keary, Kerrey, Kerrie

Kevin *Ir. Gael.* "Handsome" (a meaning that certainly applies
to two famous Kevins: actors Kline and Costner). Originally

an Irish name that spread to wider use in the 20th century. Most popular in the 1960s but still fairly standard.

Kevan, Keven, Kevon, Kevyn

Khalid *Arab.* "Never-ending."

Kieran *Ir. Gael.* "Dark, swarthy." Becoming popular in Ireland and showing some signs of spreading further afield.

Ciaran, Keiran, Kiernan

Killian *Ir. Gael.* "Small and fierce."

Kilean, Kilian, Killean

Kingsley *OE.* Place name: "king's meadow." Surname transferred to first name, particularly in Britain.

Kingsly, Kinsey, Kinsley

Kirby *OE.* Place name: "church village." Mostly 19th-century use.

Kerbey, Kerbie, Kirbey, Kirbie, Kirkby

Kirk *ONorse.* "Church." Some 19th-century use in Britain, but it was really brought into circulation by actor Kirk Douglas.

Kerk, Kirke

Kit Diminutive of **Christopher** (*Gk.* "Bearer of Christ"). A nickname for Christopher long before **Chris** was thought of. Christopher Columbus named the Caribbean island of Saint Kitts for himself and Saint Christopher, the patron saint of travelers.

Kitt

Kurt *Ger.* Variation of **Conrad** (*OG.* "Courageous advice").

Kyle *Scot.* Place name: "narrow spit of land." Well-traveled parents may have crossed the Kyle of Lochalsh to reach the Isle of Skye. Kyle was most popular in 1990, but use has slackened. A feminine version of the name, **Kylie,** is gaining popularity.

Laird *Scot.* "Lord of the land."

Lance Variation of **Lancelot.** Mildly popular on its own from the mid-20th century.
> **Lantz, Lanz, Launce**

Lancelot *OF.* "Servant." Most famous, of course, for the knight of the Round Table who seduced King Arthur's wife, Guinevere. Used as a first name in the romantic 19th century, rare for the last fifty years.
> **Launcelot**

Landon *OE.* Place name: "grassy plain."
> **Land, Landan, Landen, Landin**

Langdon *OE.* Place name: "long hill."
> **Landon, Langden**

Larkin *Ir. Gael.* "Rough, fierce."

Larry Diminutive of **Lawrence.** Given as an independent name in the 20th century and with some regularity today.

Lawford *OE.* Place name: "the hill ford."

Lawrence *Lat.* "From Laurentium." Laurentium was a city south of Rome known for its numerous laurel trees. Though the place no longer exists, the name endures, at first given staying power by the popularity of Saint Lawrence (who was martyred by being grilled alive). Brought to Britain with the Norman Conquest, revived in the United States in the 20th century.

> **Larenz, Larry, Lars, Laurance, Laurence, Laurens, Laurent, Laurentius, Loren, Lorenz, Lorenzo, Lorin**

Lee *OE.* Place name: "pasture or meadow." One of the few truly unisex names. Usually a name becomes primarily feminine once it is used for girls (**Ashley, Leslie**). The tenacious masculine hold on Lee may have been helped by tough-guy actor Lee Marvin. American use, peaking in the 1950s, seems to have been sparked by admiration for Confederate General Robert E. Lee.

> **Lea, Leigh**

Leo *Lat.* "Lion." Common in Roman times and the name of 13 popes, but it was infrequently used in the 18th and early 19th centuries. Astrological appeal notwithstanding, it is only moderately used today.

> **Lee, Leon, Leonel, Lev, Lyon**

Leonard *OG.* "Lion-bold." Name of a saint who was much venerated in the Middle Ages (as patron of prisoners, among others), but it did not inspire many parents until the

18th century. Use grew gradually to 1930 and has diminished since then.

Len, Lenard, Lennart, Leonhard, Leonid

Leroy *OF.* "The king." Occupational name: one of the servants or pages of a king. Revived in the late 19th century, especially in the United States, but use today is minimal.

Elroi, Elroy, Leroi, Roy

Lester *OE.* Place name: "from Leicester," an area in central England. First-name use dates from the mid-19th century, and its popularity lasted about a hundred years.

Leicester, Les

Levi *Heb.* "Joined, attached." In the Old Testament, one of Jacob's sons, whose descendants (known as the Levites) were Israel's tribe of priests.

Levin, Levon, Levy

Lewis Anglicization of **Louis** (*OG./OF.* "Renowned warrior"). Briefly popular in the late 19th century but now takes a back seat to Louis.

Lew, Lewes, Lou, Louis

Liam *Ir.* Variation of **William** (*OG.* "Will-helmet"). Use has increased since 1990.

Lincoln *OE.* Place name: "town by the pool." Surname transferred occasionally to a first name. The fame of Abraham Lincoln did not, surprisingly enough, encourage parents to use the name widely.

Linc, Link

Linus *Gk.* "Flax." May have originated as a descriptive name, applied to someone with flaxen or extremely pale hair. This description does not relate to today's best-known Linus, the famous *Peanuts* character who is lost without his blanket.

> Lino

Lionel *Lat.* "Young lion." Used in the Middle Ages and never resoundingly revived beyond a twinge of popularity in the 1920s and 1930s.

> Leonello, Lionell, Lyonel

Logan *Ir. Gael.* Place name: "small hollow."

> Logen

Lorenzo *It.* Variation of **Lawrence** (*Lat.* "From Laurentium"). Used more often in the United States than Italy.

> Laurencio, Lorentz, Lorenzino

Louis *OG./Fr.* "Renowned warrior." The German form is **Ludwig**, and an early French variant was **Clovis**, a name borne by several Frankish kings. The later French kings (18 of them) who chose Louis as their name were no doubt harking back to those early monarchs, one of whom included the 13th-century saint. **Luis** is now by far the most popular form in the United States.

> Aloysius, Lew, Lewes, Lewis, Lodovico, Lou, Ludovic, Ludwig, Luigi, Luis

Lowell *OF.* "Young wolf." Mostly 19th-century use.

> Lovel, Lovell, Lowe, Lowel

Lucas Variant of **Luke.** Generally a transferred last name but gaining popularity in Britain as a first name. Quite popular in the United States as well.

    Loucas, Loukas, Lukas

Lucian *Lat.* "Light." More unusual form of **Lucius,** which itself is quite rare.

    Luciano, Lucianus, Lucien, Lukyan

Lucius *Lat.* "Light." Used by the Romans but extremely scarce in the 20th century.

    Luca, Lucas, Lucias, Lucio, Lukas, Luke, Lukeus

Ludwig *Ger.* "Renowned in battle." Very unusual in English-speaking countries, where **Louis** or **Lewis** are used instead.

    Ludo, Ludovic, Ludovico

Luke *Gk.* "From Lucanus," a region of southern Italy. Not, strictly speaking, a nickname for **Lucius** and **Lucian,** though it may be used that way. The most famous Luke is, of course, the author of the Gospel and of Acts. He was a physician, and is patron saint of doctors and artists. After medieval use, rather neglected, but the name is turning up quite frequently in preschools and hospital nurseries.

    Loukas, Luc, Lucas, Lucian, Lucien, Lucio, Lucius, Lukas

Luther *OG.* "Army people." Generally homage to Martin Luther, the German religious reformer, or to Martin Luther King Jr., the civil rights activist.

    Lotario, Lothair, Lothar, Lothario, Louther, Lutero

Lyle *OF.* Place name: "the island." First-name use was mostly in the middle of the 20th century.

> **Lisle, Lyall, Lyell, Lysle**

Lyman *OE.* "Meadow dweller."

> **Leaman, Leyman**

Lyndon *OE.* Place name: "linden tree hill." First-name use coincides with the 19th-century fondness for transferred surnames, but it has been given extra renown by President Lyndon Baines Johnson.

> **Lin, Linden, Lindon, Lindy, Lyn, Lynden**

Mac *Scot. Gael.* "Son of." Also used as a nickname for given names that begin with "Mac-," many of which are transferred last names.

> **Mack, Mackey, Mackie**

Maddox *Anglo-Welsh.* "Benefactor's son."

> **Maddocks, Madocks, Madox**

Malachi *Heb.* "Angel, messenger." Name of one of the minor prophets in the Old Testament but not widely used.

> **Malachy, Malechy**

Malcolm *Scot. Gael.* "Devotee of St. Columba." The name of the prince of Scotland who became king after Macbeth murdered his father, Duncan. (Shakespeare's play was based on historical fact.) The name has been used primarily in Scotland, but it spread more widely in the middle of the 20th century.

Malcolum, Malkolm

Malik *Arab.* "Master."

Maleek, Maliq

Manfred *OE.* "Man of peace." Seldom found in real life but used by Byron for an antihero in an eponymous epic poem.

Manfredo, Manfried

Manuel Diminutive of **Emanuel** (*Heb.* "God be with us"). Most widely used in Spanish-speaking countries, but it has a considerable presence in the United States as well.

Mano, Manolo, Manny

Marcel *Fr.* Diminutive of **Marcellus** (*Lat.* "Little warrior"). One of the less common of a group of names that all have their root in the Roman god of war, Mars.

Marceau, Marcello, Marcellus

Marcus *Lat.* "Warlike." The root of such names as **Mark** and **Marcel** based on the name of the Roman war god, Mars. Common enough in Roman times but unknown in English-speaking countries until the 19th century.

Marc, Marco, Markus

Mark *Lat.* "Warlike." The anglicized version of **Marcus** and the most popular in the United States. In spite of the automatic exposure given to the name by the evangelist Saint Mark, it was not widely used in the Middle Ages, nor indeed was it really common until a sudden inexplicable flurry of use in the 1950s.

Marc, Marco, Marcos, Marcus, Mario, Marius, Marko

Marlon *OF.* "Little hawk," or possibly a variation of **Merlin.** Current use, which is scanty, is inspired by the career of actor Marlon Brando.

Marlin

Marshall *OF.* Occupational name: "horse-keeper." Also a military title of great honor, as in "field marshal." As a last name, common in Scotland. Used rather widely as a first name since the early 19th century.

Marschal, Marsh, Marshal

Martin *Lat.* "Warlike." Like **Marcus** and its variants, Martin originates with the Roman war god, Mars. The 4th-century Saint Martin (most famous for dividing his cloak in two and giving half to a beggar) was much venerated, making his name popular in the Middle Ages. The influence of Protestant reformer Martin Luther may have added to the name's appeal, since it was used very steadily right into the 19th century, though there are comparatively few variants.

Martell, Marten, Martijn, Martinos, Martyn

Marvin Origin obscure, though many sources suggest Old

English for "sea lover," while others claim that it is Welsh. Popular in the United States starting in the 19th century, peaking in the 1920s, and now unusual.

Marven, Marwin, Mervin

Mason *OF.* Occupational name: "stoneworker." Transferred from surname status starting in the mid-19th century.

Matthew *Heb.* "Gift of the Lord." Like **John, Luke,** and **Mark,** given great exposure by the author of one of the four Gospels. In more religious eras, parents would hear these names over and over again in the course of a year. Matthew began to be neglected in the 19th century and was infrequently used early in the 20th until an enthusiastic revival at midcentury. It has been one of the top five names in the United States since 1981.

Mateo, Mathew, Mathias, Mathieu, Mats, Matt, Matthias

Maurice *Lat.* "Dark-skinned, Moorish." Roman name brought to Britain by the Normans and widely used into the 17th century. A 19th-century revival faded around 1900, but the name still occurs.

Mauricio, Maurits, Maurizio, Morey, Moritz, Morris, Mo

Max Diminutive of **Maximilian** and **Maxwell.** Appeared at the turn of the 20th century, fashionable by the 1930s, then faded, but today's parents are showing interest in it again.

Maks, Maxence, Maxson

Maximilian *Lat.* "Greatest." Appropriately enough, used
by the emperor of Mexico and the Holy Roman emperor,
though a bit of a mouthful for a child.

> **Mac, Maks, Maksim, Massimo, Max, Maxime,
> Maximiliano, Maximo**

Maxwell *OE.* Place name: maybe "Maccus's well," though
some sources also suggest "large well" or "important
man's well." Mostly Scottish last name, fairly common as
a first name.

Melvin Could come from a number of sources: possibly Irish
Gaelic for "polished chief," Old English for "sword friend,"
or an adaptation of **Melville.**

> **Mel, Melvyn**

Menachem *Heb.* "Comforter."

> **Menahem, Nachum, Nahum**

Mendel *Semitic.* "Wisdom, learning."

> **Mendeley, Mendell**

Mercer *ME.* Occupational name: "storekeeper."

> **Merce**

Merlin *ME.* "Small falcon." Also the name (via a mistransla-
tion: *see also* **Mervin**) of the wizard of the Arthurian legends. Use dates from the 20th century.

> **Marlin, Marlon, Merle, Merlyn, Merlynn**

Mervin *Old Welsh.* "Sea hill." **Mervyn** is more common in
Britain. Merlin, the wizard of Arthurian legend, was known

in Welsh as Myrddin, translated into Latin as **Merlin.** The
name was mildly popular around the turn of the 20th
century.

> Merven, Mervyn, Merwin, Merwyn

Micah *Heb.* Variant of **Michael.** Very easily confused with
Michael when it is spoken.

> Mike, Mikey, Mikal, Mycah

Michael *Heb.* "Who is like the Lord?" In the New Testament,
Michael is the name of the archangel who defeats the
dragon. Usage was steady until a period of neglect that
lasted from the early 19th to the early 20th century. The
subsequent revival was immense, and Michael was the
most popular name for American boys from the mid-1960s
right through to 1997, when it was displaced by **Jacob.**
Even in the 21st century, this continues to be a favorite.

> Micael, Micheal, Michel, Michele, Mickey,
> Miguel, Mihail, Mikael, Mike, Mikey, Mikhail,
> Miko, Mitchell, Mychal

Miles Several possible origins, including Latin for "soldier,"
Old German for "merciful," or variant of **Emil** (*Lat.* "Eager
to please"). Since the end of the 18th century, it has been
quite unusual.

> Milan, Milo, Myles

Miller *OE.* Occupational name. Use as a first name began in
the late 19th century, is now sparing.

> Millar, Myller

Milo *Ger.* Variation of **Miles.** Very unusual.

Milton *OE.* Place name: "mill town" or perhaps "middle town." One of the more commonplace names transferred to a first name, dating from the early 19th century.

> **Milt, Mylton**

Mitchell *ME.* Variant of **Michael.** The last name evolved in the Middle Ages, when surnames began to be regularly used, and it was transferred back to a first name in the 19th century.

> **Mitch, Mitchel**

Mohammed *Arab.* "Highly praised." *See also* **Muhammad.**

Montgomery *OE.* Place name: "mount of the rich man." Unusual as a first name and very likely to be shortened to **Monty.**

> **Montgomerie, Monty**

Mordecai *Heb.* Meaning not clear but possibly "follower of Marduk" (who was a god of the Babylonians). An Old Testament name revived by the Puritans and neglected since the 19th century.

> **Mordechai, Mordy, Mort**

Moreland *OE.* Place name: "moor land." *Moor* is a British term referring to a large, rolling expanse of scrubby, infertile wild land.

> **Moorland, Morland**

Morgan Different sources give several meanings, including

Welsh for "great and bright" and Old English for "bright or white sea dweller." Quite well used for girls in the United States.

Morgen, Morgun, Morrgan

Morley *OE.* Place name: "meadow on the moor."

Moorley, Moorly, Morlee, Morleigh, Morly, Morrley

Morris Anglicization of **Maurice** (*Lat.* "Dark-skinned, Moorish"). Now more common as a surname.

Morey, Morice, Moris, Morrey, Morrie, Morrison, Morrisson, Morry

Mortimer *OF.* Place name: "still water." Literally, "dead sea," *mort mer.* First-name use, as with so many of these place names, dates from the 19th century.

Mort, Morty, Mortymer

Morton *OE.* Place name: "moor town." Like **Mortimer,** used as a first name since the 19th century, though probably more common.

Morten

Moses History unclear. Some sources suggest Hebrew for "savior," while others claim it means "taken from the water." The latter definition clearly comes from the biblical story of the infant Moses afloat in the bulrushes, where he was rescued by Pharaoh's daughter and later became the great leader of the exiled Israelites. Always current in Jewish families, adopted by the Puritans in the 17th century, now uncommon.

Moe, Moise, Moises, Moyses

Muhammad *Arab.* "Greatly praised." Name of the prophet and founder of Islam. There are some five hundred variants of this name, and if they were all counted as one name, it would be the most popular name in the world.

Hamid, Hammad, Mahmoud, Mahomet, Mehmet, Mohamet, Mohammad, Mohammed

Murphy *Ir. Gael.* "Sea fighter." A quintessentially Irish last name in occasional use as a first name.

Murphey, Murphie

Murray *Scot. Gael.* Place name, or possibly "mariner." Somewhat common as a first name in the 1930s and 1940s but now little used.

Moray, Murrey, Murry

Nabil *Arab.* "Highborn."

Nabeel

Najib *Arab.* "Of highborn parentage."

Nagib, Najeeb

Nasser *Arab.* "The winner."
> Nasir, Naser, Nasr

Nathan *Heb.* "Given." Old Testament name revived in the
18th century and quite popular since the mid-1960s. It
has been in the top 50 boys' names in the United States
for a dozen years and cracked the top 20 in 2004.
> Nat, Natan, Nate

Nathaniel *Heb.* "Given by God." New Testament name of one
of the apostles (who was also called Bartholomew). Used
by the Puritans and a steady presence ever since, though
quite a bit less popular than **Nathan.**
> Nat, Nathanial, Nathanyel

Ned Diminutive of **Edward** (*OE.* "Wealthy defender");
Edmund (*OE.* "Wealthy protector").

Nehemiah *Heb.* "The Lord's comfort." Old Testament prophet, Puritan name, rare in the 20th and 21st centuries.
> Nechemia, Nechemiah, Nechemya

Neil *Ir. Gael.* "Champion." Although the name of the most
famous Celtic king of Ireland (Niall of the Nine Hostages),
it has been used mostly in Scotland until the middle of the
20th century.
> Neal, Neale, Neill, Neils, Nels, Nial, Niall, Niles

Nelson *Eng.* "Son of Neil." Established by parents who ad-
mired the exploits of English Admiral Nelson at the Battle
of Trafalgar. Used consistently, if never widely, since then.
> Neilson, Nelsen, Niles, Nilson

Nestor *Gk.* "Traveler, voyager."

> **Nestore, Nestorio**

Neville *OF.* Place name: "new town." More common in Britain.

> **Nevil, Nevile**

Newton *OE.* Place name: "New town." Like many place names turned last names, made the move to a first name in the 19th century and has now drifted back to last-name status.

Nicholas *Gk.* "People of victory." A New Testament name given even greater fame by the 4th-century Saint Nicholas, patron saint of children and (via his Dutch name, Sinte Klaas) the original Santa Claus. The name was widespread in the Middle Ages through the 17th century, then had a long period of disuse that ended in the middle of the 20th century. It spurted to top 10 use from 1993 to 2002 and is now a little less popular.

> **Claus, Cole, Colin, Klaes, Nic, Niccolo, Nichol, Nichols, Nick, Nickey, Nickolas, Nicol, Nicolai, Nicolls, Nik, Nikolai**

Nigel *Ir. Gael.* "Champion." Related not, as many sources claim, to the Latin *niger* ("black") but to the Latin form of **Neil,** Nigellus. Almost exclusively a British name popular in the 20th century.

Noah *Heb.* Meaning unclear, possibly "rest" or "wandering."

The latter would be appropriate for the patriarch who drifted in the ark for 40 days. Steadily but not widely used since the 17th century.

Noach, Noak, Noé

Noble *Lat.* "Aristocratic." Use as a first name may derive from surnames or from the use of the adjective as a name. Mostly 19th century.

Noel *Fr.* "Christmas." Used since the Middle Ages but not very widespread. More likely to be chosen for girls.

Nowel, Nowell

Nolan *Ir. Gael.* "Renowned." A last name transferred to first name.

Noland, Nolen, Nolin

Norman *OE.* "Northerner." The Normans of France were originally from Scandinavia, or the North, but the name was also used in England even before the Norman Conquest. After medieval use, it was neglected until a substantial 19th-century revival, which has long since faded.

Norm, Normand

Oberon *OG.* "Highborn and bearlike." This is its more famous
(though infrequently used) form, as used by Shakespeare
for the king of the Fairies in *A Midsummer Night's Dream.*
It also occurs (very rarely) as **Auberon.**

> **Auberon, Auberron, Oberron**

Octavius *Lat.* "Eighth child." In English-speaking countries
the name had its heyday in the Victorian era of large families. It has survived slightly better in Latin countries.

> **Octave, Octavian, Octavio, Ottavio**

Olaf *Scan.* "Ancestor." A royal name in Norway, as well as a
saint's name, but it did not catch on when it came to the
British Isles with Norse invaders.

> **Olaff, Olav, Ole, Olin**

Oleg *Rus.* "Holy."

Oliver *Lat.* "Olive tree" is the most common meaning as-
signed, but some scholars suggest Old Norse for "kindly"
or "ancestor," among other possibilities. It came to Britain
from France, and the controversial Lord Protector Oliver
Cromwell made it unpopular for generations. A mild revival
occurred in the late 19th century, and the name is infrequently used in the United States today. It is very fashionable in England, though.

> **Olivero, Olivier, Olivor**

Omar *Arab.* "Elevated; follower of the prophet"; *Heb.*
"Expressive."
>**Omer**

Oren *Heb.* "Pine tree"; *Ir. Gael.* "Fair, pale-skinned." Very
unusual.
>**Orin, Orren, Orrin**

Orion *Gk.* "Son of fire or light." In Greek mythology, Orion
was a mighty hunter who was turned into the constellation
of the same name.
>**Oryon**

Orlando *Sp.* Variation of **Roland** (*OG.* "Famous land").
Mostly literary and minor late 19th-century use.
>**Orland, Roland, Rolando**

Orson *Lat.* "Like a bear." In an old French story, a child
named Orson is reared in the forest by a bear. The name
is very unusual, though it may be used by ardent fans of
director Orson Welles.
>**Orsin, Orsini, Orsino, Orsis**

Orville *OF.* Place name: "town of gold." Though the name
translates this way, it may actually have been coined by an
18th-century novelist. Never widespread.
>**Orv, Orval, Orvell, Orvil**

Osbert *OE.* "Divine and bright." Anglo-Saxon name revived
mildly with the antiquarian craze of the 19th century but
now extremely rare.

Osborn *OE.* "Divine bear." The 19th-century revival of this

Anglo-Saxon name was followed by another small spurt of use in the middle of the 20th century.

Osborne, Osbourn, Osbourne, Osburn, Ozzie

Oscar *Scan.* "Divine spear." Anglo-Saxon name revived by 18th-century literary use, reaching substantial popularity by the late 19th century. Fans of *Sesame Street* might hesitate to name a baby for the curmudgeonly Oscar the Grouch, but some parents bravely persist.

Oskar, Ossie, Ozzy

Oswald *OE.* "Divine power." Another Anglo-Saxon name that endured partially because of the fame of two saints of the name. Use has been mostly 19th century, though actor Ozzie Nelson's real name was Oswald.

Ossie, Osvald, Osvaldo, Ozzie, Waldo

Otis *OE.* "Son of Otto." Use is mostly American.

Oates, Otess

Otto *OG.* "Prosperous." German name that was fairly common in English-speaking countries until Otto von Bismarck's German armies became threateningly powerful at the turn of the 20th century. The Second World War against Germany further limited the name's use.

Odo, Othello, Otho

Owen *Welsh.* Variation of **Eugene** (*Gk.* "Wellborn"). Fairly common outside Wales since the 18th century. Now steadily used in the United States.

Ewan, Ewen, Owain, Owin

Pablo *Sp.* Variation of **Paul** (*Lat.* "Little").
>   Pablos

Paco *Sp.* Variation of **Francis** (*Lat.* "From France"). A diminutive of **Francisco.**
>   Paquito

Palmer *OE.* "One who holds a palm." Usually indicates a pilgrim, who would have carried a palm branch on his pilgrimage.
>   Pallmer, Palmerston

Paris *OE.* Place name: "From Paris," the city. Also a figure in Greek mythology who was Helen of Troy's lover. Use of the name is predominantly American and is beginning to cross over to use for girls.
>   Parris

Parker *OE.* "Park keeper." Occupational name turned surname, popular in the 19th century as a given name but now more unusual.
>   Parke, Parkes, Parks

Parrish *OF.* "Ecclesiastical locality." A parish is the area under the care of one pastor or priest. The name would originally have been a last name based on a place name.
>   Parish, Parris, Parriss

Pascal *Fr.* "Child of Easter." Used as a first name in English-speaking countries only since the 1960s, and very scarce.

> Pascale, Paschal, Pasquale

Patrick *Lat.* "Noble, patrician." A Roman name made famous by the 5th-century missionary (and patron of Ireland) Saint Patrick, whose feast day on March 17 is celebrated with parades in the United States, an honor accorded to few other saints. The name spread outside of Ireland in the 18th century and was widely used by the middle of the 20th century. It is now steadily used and has lost its firm associations with Ireland.

> Paddy, Padhraig, Padraic, Pat, Patric, Patricio, Patrizio

Paul *Lat.* "Small." Popular Roman and medieval name whose tremendously widespread modern use dates from the 18th century. Paul is the name of the resilient Sir Paul McCartney, as well of the pope who spearheaded Vatican II. It is not fashionable in the current vogue for original names; in fact, use has declined steadily since the mid-1960s.

> Paavo, Pablo, Paolo, Paulus, Pauly, Pavel

Pedro *Sp.* Variant of **Peter** (*Gk.* "Rock").

> Pedrio, Pepe, Petrolino, Piero

Percy *Fr.* "From Percy." A Norman place name that became associated with an immensely powerful aristocratic family in the north of England.

> Pearcy, Percey, Percie

Peregrine *Lat.* "Traveler, pilgrim." *Peregrinations* is a synonym for "wanderings." Peregrine is also the name of a kind of falcon. The name persists in a small way in Britain.

> **Peregrin, Peregrino, Peregryn**

Peter *Gk.* "Rock." New Testament name; the saint who, tradition has it, guards the gates to Heaven. The name's greatest popularity came in the first three-quarters of the twentieth century, prompted, some sources suggest, by the play *Peter Pan.*

> **Peadar, Pearce, Peder, Pedro, Peirce, Per, Perkin, Perry, Pete, Petr, Piero, Pierre, Pierson, Piet, Pieter, Pietro, Piotr**

Peyton *OE.* Place name: "fighting man's estate." Primarily American use, probably as a transferred last name—that is, a mother's maiden name.

> **Payton**

Philip *Gk.* "Lover of horses." The name of one of the 12 apostles and a staple since early Christian times, though it receded somewhat in the 19th century. A 20th-century resurgence peaked in the 1960s, and like **Peter,** Philip is familiar but not common.

> **Felipe, Filip, Filippo, Phelps, Phil, Philippe, Philippos, Phillip, Phillips**

Philo *Gk.* "Loving."

Phineas Derivation and meaning unknown, though many

sources offer Hebrew for "oracle." Another possible
meaning is "mouth of brass," which would be appropriate
for showman Phineas T. Barnum.

> Fineas, Phinnaeus, Pinchas

Pierce Variation of **Peter** (*Gk.* "Rock"). One of a group of
Peter-derived names along with **Pearson, Piers,** and
so on.

> Pearce, Pears, Pearson, Peirce, Piers, Pierson,
> Piersson

Piers *Gk.* "Rock." **Peter** is actually the Latin form of the name
that the Normans took to Britain as Piers. This form, along
with **Pierce,** has been an alternate form more popular in
Britain than in the United States.

> Pearce, Pears, Pearson, Pierce, Pierson,
> Piersson

Pomeroy *OF.* Place name: "apple orchard." The French word
for apple is *pomme.*

> Pommeray, Pommeroy

Porter *Lat.* "Gatekeeper." Occupational name.

Powell *OE.* Surname related to **Paul.**

> Powel

Prentice *ME.* "Apprentice."

> Prentis, Prentiss

Prescott *OE.* Place name: "priest's cottage."

> Prescot, Prestcot, Prestcott

Presley *OE*. Place name: "priest's meadow." In the Middle
Ages, when these names came into use, the priest was a
very important figure in any community. Of course, today
the name is associated with another important figure, Elvis
Presley.

> **Presleigh, Presly, Presslee, Pressley, Prestley,
> Priestley, Priestly**

Preston *OE*. Place name: "priest's estate."

Primo *It*. "First; firstborn." Primo may allude to great pride in
the firstborn, especially a son.

> **Preemo, Premo, Prime**

Prince *Lat*. "Prince." As a last name, it may have indicated
someone who worked in a prince's household, and occasional first-name use is generally transferred from the
last name.

> **Printze, Prinz, Prinze**

Proctor *Lat*. "Official, administrator." Occupational last name.

> **Prockter, Procter**

Prosper *Lat*. "Fortunate," as in "prosperous."

> **Prospero**

Pryor *Lat*. "Monastic leader." A prior is the monk in charge
of a monastery, so this might be an occupational name.
However, the tradition of monastic chastity would seem to
prevent this name from being handed down to children.

> **Prior**

Quentin *Lat.* "Fifth." Probably used without any consideration of its meaning, since so few families extend to five children these days.

    Quenton, Quint, Quintin, Quintus

Quincy *OF.* Place name: "estate of the fifth son." Last name of a prominent Massachusetts family whose name is borne by a town and by the sixth U.S. president, John Quincy Adams.

    Quin, Quincey, Quinsy

Quinn *Ir. Gael.* Meaning unknown. Very common Irish last name occasionally transferred to first-name status, especially in the United States.

Rafi *Arab.* "Holding high."

    Rafee, Raffi, Raffy

Raleigh *OE.* Place name: "meadow of roe deer." Commemorates Sir Walter Raleigh, explorer and court favorite of Queen Elizabeth I, who is supposed to have

spread his cape over a puddle so that she could cross with
dry feet. The city in North Carolina was named for him.

Ralegh, Rawleigh, Rawley, Rawly

Ralph *OE.* "Wolf counsel." A name that has been steadily, if
not enormously, popular for the last thousand years. Its
greatest vogue in the United States occurred at the turn of
the 19th century.

Rafe, Ralf, Raoul, Rolf, Rolph

Ramon *Sp.* Variation of **Raymond** (*OG.* "Counselor-protector"). Given its greatest exposure by the silent-movie star
of the 1920s, Ramon Novarro.

Ramsay *OE.* Place name: "raven island" or "ram island."
Originally a last name common in Scotland.

Ramsey

Randall *OE.* "Shield wolf." This is the medieval spoken form
of **Randolph.** Enjoyed some popularity with parents in the
baby boom era.

Randal, Randell, Randle, Randy

Randolph *OE.* "Shield wolf." From the same root as
Randall, which has been more popular in the United
States.

Randolf, Randy

Raoul *Fr.* Variant of **Ralph** (*OE.* "Wolf counsel"). Uncommon
among English-speaking parents.

Raul, Roul

Raphael *Heb.* "God has healed." The name of one of the archangels, possibly (because of his name) the one who stirred the waters at the pool of Bethesda to give it healing powers. Most common in very religious eras (16th and 17th centuries) and the 19th century, which cherished the picturesque.

> Rafael, Rafaelle, Rafaello, Rafal, Rafe, Rafel, Rafello

Rashid *Arab.* "Righteous, rightly advised." **Rashida** is also used for girls.

> Rasheed, Rasheid, Rasheyd

Rawlins *OF.* Ultimately a diminutive of **Roland**.

> Rawlinson, Rawson

Raymond *OG.* "Counselor-protector." Old Teutonic name that was used in the Middle Ages, then forgotten until a very strong 19th-century revival, especially in the United States. Though far from fashionable, it is steadily used.

> Raimondo, Raimund, Ramon, Ramone, Ray, Raymondo, Raymundo

Read *OE.* "Red-haired." Descriptive name that long ago became a last name and then a first name, especially in the United States.

> Reade, Reed, Reid

Reginald *OE.* "Counsel power." **Ronald** and **Reynolds** are just two of the names that come from the same source;

Reginald's popularity was mainly British and 19th century.

Naldo, Rainault, Raynald, Reg, Reggie, Reinald, Reinhold, Renaud, Renault, Reynaldo, Rinaldo, Ronald

Remus *Lat.* "Swift." The name of one of the legendary twins (the other was Romulus) who founded Rome.

Remo

Remy *Fr.* "From Rheims." Champagne and the fine brandies made from champagne are the principal products of Rheims, a town in central France. The name is used, albeit rarely, for both boys and girls.

Remey, Remie, Remmy

René *Fr.* "Reborn." The modern form of **Renatus,** which did not survive as a male name. Unlike the female version, René has not really spread beyond French-speaking families, probably because it is well entrenched as a girl's name.

Renat, Renato, Renatus

Renny *Ir. Gael.* "Small and mighty."

Renzo Diminutive of **Lorenzo** (*Lat.* "Laurel").

Reuben *Heb.* "Behold, a son." Old Testament name that came into general use in the 18th century.

Reuven, Ruben, Rubin, Rubino

Rex *Lat.* "King." Mostly 20th-century use, possibly influenced by actor Rex Harrison.

Reynolds Variant of **Reginald** (*OE.* "Counsel power").
Probably most familiar in the United States as a surname,
though in the Middle Ages this was the most common
form of **Reginald**.
> Reynaldo, Reynold, Rinaldo

Rhys *Welsh.* "Fiery, zealous." This is the native Welsh form
of the name that appears more often in English-speaking
countries as **Reece.** It is currently very popular in Wales.
> Reece, Rees

Richard *OG.* "Dominant ruler." Norman name that went on to
be a steady favorite for the last nine hundred years, with
one century (the 19th) of neglect. In the current hunger
for the unusual, it is somewhat overlooked, but plenty of
parents still choose it.
> Dick, Dicky, Ric, Ricardo, Rich, Rick, Ricky, Rico,
> Ritchie

Rick Diminutive of **Frederick** and **Richard.** Used independently, though more common as a nickname.
> Ric, Rickey, Rickie, Ricky, Rik

Ridley *OE.* Place name: "Red meadow."
> Riddley, Ridlea, Ridleigh, Ridly

Riley *Ir. Gael.* "Courageous." Irish last name used as a first
name since the mid-1800s.
> Reilly, Ryley

Ripley *OE.* Place name: "shouting man's meadow."
> Ripleigh, Riply

Rob Diminutive of **Robert.** The most common nickname for Robert is probably **Bob,** but Rob may be given more often as an independent name.

> **Robb, Robbie, Robby**

Robert *OE.* "Bright fame." Another staple male name common for the last millennium and still in the American top 50. It has steadily drifted out of top 10 status since 1989.

> **Bert, Bob, Bobby, Rab, Rob, Robbins, Robby, Roberto, Robertson, Robin, Robinson, Robson, Robyn, Rupert, Ruprecht**

Rocco *Ger./It.* "Rest." The most common American form of the name of a popular saint who cured plague victims. He was especially venerated in Italy, which may be why this version of the name is the most common. **Rocky** is usually a nickname.

> **Roch, Roche, Rocko, Rocky**

Rockwell *OE.* Place name: "rock spring."

Roderick *OG.* "Renowned rule." Most commonly used in Scotland and other parts of Britain; never a great favorite in America.

> **Broderick, Brodrick, Rhodric, Rod, Roddrick, Roddy, Roderic, Roderigo, Rodrick, Rodrigo, Rodrigues, Rodriquez, Rodryk, Roric Rory**

Rodney *OE.* Place name: "island near the clearing." Like many last names, this one began intensive use as a first

name in the mid-19th century. This mild popularity has
endured since the 1850s.

Rodnee, Rodnie

Rogan *Ir. Gael.* "Redhead." Irish Gaelic has several names to
indicate red hair; but then, the Irish people produce many
redheads.

Roger *OG.* "Renowned spearman." At its most popular in the
Middle Ages and the 19th and 20th centuries, but on the
wane since the 1950s.

**Dodge, Rodger, Rogelio, Rogerio, Rogers,
Rogiero, Ruggero, Ruggiero, Rutger**

Roland *OG.* "Renowned land." **Orlando** is a more common
variant in several European languages. For a long time,
Rowland was the preferred version in English. The name
dates from the Dark Ages, and the most famous Roland
was the valorous nephew of Charlemagne, about whom
many romantic tales were written.

Orlando, Rolando, Roldan, Rollin, Rollo, Rowland

Roman *Lat.* "From Rome." The name of several obscure
saints and one short-lived pope. The significance of the
name no doubt comes from the fact that Rome is the
center of the Roman Catholic faith.

Romain, Romaine, Romano, Romanos

Romeo *It.* "Pilgrim to Rome." Cannot be used without reference to the famous romance, so it is sure to engender a
lot of teasing.

Romulus *Lat.* "Man of Rome." Along with Remus, the legendary founder of Rome, though Romulus actually murdered his twin brother in a quarrel over where to situate the city, which he then ruled for 37 years.

Romolo

Ronald *OE.* "Counsel power." Though it was fairly common in the 1940s and 1950s, most parents will associate Ronald with two-term president Ronald Reagan and with clown Ronald McDonald. In spite of these uncool connections, the name is used from time to time.

Renaldo, Ron, Ronaldo, Ronnie

Ronan *Ir. Gael.* "Little seal." Mostly Irish use.

Rory *Ir. Gael.* "Red." Also occurs as a nickname for **Roderick.** Mostly Scottish use, but the name seems highly eligible for 21st-century popularity, since it is unusual without being weird.

Rosario *Port.* "The rosary." Most common, for obvious reasons, among Catholic families.

Roscoe *ONorse.* Place name: "woods of the female deer."

Ross, Rosscoe

Ross *Scot. Gael.* "Headland." A place name in Scotland and very popular as a first name there, as well. The name (like so many of the "R" names) may also come from the Gaelic word for "red."

Rosse, Rossell

Rowan *OE.* Place name: "rowan tree." Also possibly another Gaelic name meaning "red." Presumably, since the term applied to so many people, variations in the name were necessary to tell them apart.

Roan, Rohan, Rowe

Roy *Ir. Gael./Gael.* "Red"; *Fr.* "King." Most popular early in the 20th century.

Rey, Roi, Ruy

Rudolph *OG.* "Famous wolf." Parents would have to have very strong feelings about the name to use it, given the enormous fame of Rudolph the red-nosed reindeer.

Dolph, Raoul, Rodolfo, Rolf, Rudie, Rudolf, Rudy

Rufus *Lat.* "Red-haired." Another redhead name, though this one comes from Latin rather than Gaelic. Most common in the 19th century.

Ruffus, Rufous

Rupert Variation of **Robert.** Well established in Britain since the 18th century but less used in the United States.

Ruprecht

Russell *Fr.* "Redhead; red-skinned." Originally a last name but popular as a first name in the middle of the 20th century. Like most fashions of that era, the name is now somewhat neglected.

Roussell, Russ, Russel

Ryan *Irish last name.* Meaning is unclear, though some

sources connect it with "king." Has been very popular in
recent years, especially in Scotland and Ireland.

   Rian, Rien, Ryen, Ryon, Ryun

Ryder *OE.* "Horseman." Likely to be a transferred last name;
for instance, a mother's maiden name.

   Rider

Ryland *OE.* Place name: "land where rye is grown."

   Ryeland

Sabin *Lat.* "Sabine." The Sabines were a tribe living in central
Italy around the time Romulus and Remus established the
city of Rome. In an effort to provide wives for the citizens
of Rome, Romulus arranged the mass kidnapping of the
Sabine women. The name is more common in the feminine form, **Sabina**.

   Saban, Sabino, Savin

Sacha *Rus.* Diminutive of **Alexander** (*Gk.* "Defender of mankind"). Cropped up in English-speaking countries since
the 1980s. The "-a" ending in Russian is not necessarily
feminine.

   Sascha, Sasha

Said *Arab.* "Happy."

> Saeed, Sayeed, Sayid

Salim *Arab.* "Tranquility."

> Saleem, Salem, Selim

Salvatore *It.* "Savior." Used mostly by families of Latin descent.

> Sal, Salvador, Salvator

Samson *Heb.* "Sun." In the Old Testament, Samson was the warrior whose strength ebbed away when his hair was cut by Delilah. The name was used in the Middle Ages, and the Puritans kept it current with their fondness for Old Testament names, but it has not been fashionable for several hundred years.

> Sam, Sampson, Sanson

Samuel *Heb.* "Told by God." A judge and prophet in early Israel; two Old Testament books are named for him. Predictably, the name was used by the Puritans and has never really faded since then, though it peaked in the 19th century.

> Sam, Sammie, Samuele, Shem, Shmuel

Sanders *ME.* "Son of Alexander." (*Gk.* "Defender of mankind.")

> Sanderson, Sandros, Saunders, Saunderson

Sandy Diminutive of **Alexander** (*Gk.* "Defender of mankind"). Sometimes also given as a nickname based on a person's coloring.

> Sandey, Sandie, Sandino

Saul *Heb.* "Asked for." The name of the first king of Israel and also the name of the apostle Paul before his conversion to Christianity. Overlooked in the 16th-century revival of Old Testament names, at its peak in the late 19th century.
> **Shaul, Sol, Sollie**

Schuyler *Dutch.* "Shield, protection" or "scholar." Harks back to the Dutch settlers who brought the name to America in the 17th century. **Skyler** is the most popular form.
> **Schuylar, Skylar, Skyler**

Scott *OE.* "Scotsman." Use is emphatically 20th century. While the name is not fashionable, it certainly is familiar.
> **Scot, Scottie, Scotto, Scotty**

Seamus *Ir.* Variant of **James** (*Heb.* "He who supplants"). "Shamus" is old-fashioned American slang for a detective, possibly because the urban police force has traditionally been heavily Irish.
> **Seumas, Seumus, Shamus**

Sean *Ir.* Variant of **John** (*Heb.* "God is gracious"). Spread outside of Ireland only in the 20th century. Quite heavily used now, perhaps influenced by the popularity of actors Sean Connery and Sean Penn.
> **Shane, Shaughn, Shaun, Shawn**

Sebastian *Lat.* "From Sebastia" (an ancient city). Saint Sebastian, an early Christian martyr, was killed in a hail of arrows and was a favorite subject for old master painters.

The name has never been common, though the British have used it somewhat since the 1940s.

Bastian, Bastien, Seb, Sebastiano, Sebastien

Selwyn *OE.* "Manor friend." Alternatively, an offshoot of **Silvanus.** Mostly 19th-century use.

Selwin, Selwinn, Selwynn

Sergio *Lat.* "Servant, attendant." Strongly associated with Russia, perhaps because of composers Rachmaninoff and Prokofiev, yet it comes from a Latin name and was used by an early pope. This Spanish form is the most common one in the United States.

Seargeoh, Serge, Sergei, Sergey, Sergi, Sergios

Seth *Heb.* "Set, appointed." In the Old Testament, Adam and Eve's third son (after Cain and Abel). Passed over in the Puritan revival of biblical names but included to some extent in the late 20th-century revival of the same.

Seymour *OF.* "From Saint Maur." Indicates an ancestor who came from a village called Saint Maur, most probably in Normandy. Quite a popular name in the 19th century but virtually invisible today.

Seymore

Shakil *Arab.* "Good-looking, well developed." The root of Shaquille O'Neal's name, and more accurate than his parents could ever have predicted.

Shakeel, Shakill, Shaquil, Shaquille

Shalom *Heb.* "Peace." Related to **Solomon.**
> Sholom, Solomon

Shane Variant of **Sean** (*Ir.* Variant of **John.** *Heb.* "The Lord is gracious"). Popularity in the 1950s and 1960s probably depended on the film *Shane.* Now losing ground.
> Shaine, Shayn, Shayne

Sharif *Arab.* "Honest." Actor Omar Sharif.
> Shareef

Shelby *OE.* Place name: "village on the ledge."
> Shelbey, Shelbie

Sheldon *OE.* Place name: "steep valley" or possibly "flat-topped hill." Most common in the middle of the 20th century.
> Shelden, Sheldin

Shepherd *OE.* Occupational name: "shepherd." Mostly 19th-century use, very uncommon now.
> Shep, Shepard, Shephard, Sheppard

Sheridan *Ir. Gael.* Unclear meaning, possibly "wild man." Used mostly in Britain.
> Sheredan, Sheridon, Sherridan

Sherman *OE.* Occupational name: "shear man." Around the time when last names were coming into being, England's great export was wool. The wool business has given the modern world a number of other occupational names, such as **Fuller, Shepherd,** and **Weaver.**
> Scherman, Schermann, Shearman, Shermann

Sherwin *ME.* "Bright friend."

    Sherwinn, Sherwyn, Sherwynne

Sherwood *OE.* Place name: "shining forest." Sherwood Forest, a real forest in central England, was the home of the legendary bandit/hero Robin Hood.

    Sherwoode

Shlomo *Variation of* **Solomon** (*Heb.* "Peaceable").

    Shelomi, Shelomo, Shlomi

Sidney *OE.* "From Saint Denis." Famous English last name turned first name in the 18th century, very fashionable in the late 19th century, and now infrequently used for boys.

    Sid, Sydney

Siegfried *OG.* "Victory peace." The hero of the last two of Wagner's *Ring* cycle of operas, son of Siegmund, husband of Brunhilde.

Sigmund *OG.* "Victorious protector." Another character from the *Ring* cycle, son of the god Wotan. He fathers Siegfried on his own sister, Sieglinde. The other famous Sigmund is the father of psychoanalysis, Sigmund Freud. A name with many weighty connotations.

    Siegmund, Sigismond, Sigismund, Sigismundo

Silas A contraction of **Silvanus.** New Testament name used in the Puritan era and occurring since then. Has an old-fashioned air that may appeal to parents of the 21st century.

    Silvan, Silvano, Silvanus, Silvio, Sylvan

Silvanus *Lat.* "Wood dweller." Also a New Testament name
but never as widely adopted as its spinoff, **Silas.**
> Silvain, Silvano, Silvio

Silvester *Lat.* "Wooded." Original form of the name we know
as **Sylvester.**
> Silvestre, Silvestro, Sylvester

Simon *Heb.* "Listening intently." Prominent New Testament
name, one of the 12 apostles. A common name from the
Middle Ages through the 18th century, then revived early
in the 20th century. To Americans, it has a rather English
air. **Simeon,** the Old Testament version, has never been
as common.
> Shimon, Simeon, Simmonds, Simms, Simone,
> Simpson

Socrates *Gk.* Meaning unknown. The name of the great
Greek philosopher, used mostly by Greek families.
> Sokrates

Solomon *Heb.* "Peaceable." In the Old Testament, the wise
king of Israel. Used in the Middle Ages and the 18th century but currently not a common choice.
> Salomon, Salomone, Sol

Spencer *ME.* Occupational name: "provisioner." Used for
the person in a large household who dispensed food and
drink. Usually a last name but occurs as a first name, more
commonly in Britain.
> Spence, Spenser

Stacy Diminutive of **Eustace** (*Gk.* "Fertile"). More common as a female name.

> **Stacey, Stacie**

Stanislaus *Slavic.* Possibly "glorious camp or stand." The patron saint of Poland, Saint Stanislaus, was an 11th-century bishop and martyr.

> **Stanislas**

Stanley *OE.* Place name: "stony field." It is not clear why some place names, such as **Sidney** and Stanley, became popular enough that they made the transition to common first names, whereas others remain primarily last names.

> **Stan, Stanly**

Stephen *Gk.* "Crowned." As the name of Christianity's first martyr (Saint Stephen, who was stoned to death), common until the late 18th century. A slow decline was reversed in the middle of the 20th century, and **Steven** is still going very strong after a long period of great popularity. Though the "-ph-" spelling is traditional, the "-v-" is more common.

> **Esteban, Estefan, Etienne, Stefan, Stefano, Stephan, Stephens, Steve, Steven, Stevenson, Stevie**

Sterling *OE.* "Genuine, first-rate." As in sterling silver.

> **Stirling**

Stuart *OE.* Occupational name: "steward." The steward would administer a large feudal household. This was the name of kings of Scotland and England, often considered the most romantic ruling family. (Long curls, a taste for luxury, a reputation for womanizing, and a couple of beheadings all added to the romance.) Most popular in the middle of the 20th century.

Steward, Stewart

Sulaiman *Arab.* "Peaceable." The Arabic version of **Solomon.** The Turkish sultan Suleiman the Magnificent brought civilization in his country to new heights, but contemporaneous Western rulers would never have characterized him as living up to his name.

Suleiman, Suleyman

Sylvester *Lat.* "Wooded." In spite of a distinguished past, the name is now associated with a cartoon cat and an extremely muscular actor, Sylvester Stallone.

Silvester, Sly

Tad Diminutive of **Thaddeus** (meaning unknown). Also *Old Welsh.* "Father." Also used as a nickname in the United States, where "tad" is slang for "small," probably from "tadpole."

Tadd, Tadeo, Thad

Tahir *Arab.* "Pure, unsullied."

    Taheer

Tal *Heb.* "Rain, dew."

    Tahl, Talor

Tanner *OE.* Occupational name: "leather tanner." Hides need to be tanned, or treated with a substance containing tannin, before they become leather. Fairly well used, though its popularity has been waning since the late 1990s.

    Tan, Tanier, Tannen

Taylor *ME.* Occupational name: "tailor." Like many occupational names, this was first used as a given name in the 19th century. It has recently become much more popular. In the mid-1990s, it was a top 10 girls' name, which may have disqualified it as a choice for boys.

    Tailer, Tailor, Tayler

Ted Diminutive of **Theodore** (*Gk.* "Gift of God") or **Edward** (*OE.* "Wealthy defender"). Rarely used as an independent name. Parents tend to give the longer rather than the shorter version of a name, even if they have decided ahead of time to use the diminutive form.

    Tedd, Teddie, Teddy

Tennessee Cherokee place name used for the state. Made famous by playwright Tennessee Williams (whose given name was Thomas) and likely to be used by parents in homage, or perhaps in nostalgia for a childhood home.

Tennyson *ME.* "Son of Dennis." Used by 19th-century parents in homage to British poet laureate Alfred, Lord Tennyson.

> **Tenny**

Terence *Lat.* Clan name of unknown meaning, though some sources propose "smooth" or "polished." Early Christian name that was never widely adopted until the late 19th century, and even then it did not become a standard choice. The most common spelling today is **Terrance.**

> **Terencio, Terrance, Terrence, Terronce, Terry**

Terrell *OG.* "Following Thor." Thor, the god of thunder, was a crucial figure in Norse mythology. The son of Odin, the chief god, Thor was the benevolent intercessor for mankind. His name is an element in many names that have come down to us, the most notable being "Thursday."

> **Tarrall, Terrall, Terrel, Terrill**

Thaddeus *Aramaic.* Meaning unclear, though "courageous" and "praise" have been suggested. He was one of the more obscure of the 12 apostles, but even this distinction has not popularized the name.

> **Tad, Tadd, Taddeusz, Tadeo, Tadzio, Thad, Thaddaeus, Thaddaus, Thadeus**

Theodore *Gk.* "Gift of God." Early Christian name and saint's name, but it was only mildly popular until President Theodore Roosevelt brought it to prominence. (The teddy bear, of course, is named for him.) The name is now neither popular nor unpopular.

Fedor, Feodor, Fyodor, Ted, Teddy, Teodoro, Theo, Theodosius

Theodoric *OG.* "People's ruler." This is the original form of **Dietrich** and the more common **Derek** or **Dirk**. In this version it is extremely rare.

Derek, Derrick, Dieter, Dietrich, Dirck, Dirk, Rick, Ted, Teodorico

Thomas *Aramaic.* "Twin." One of the apostles was known as Doubting Thomas because he refused to recognize the risen Christ unless he could see and feel the marks of the crucifixion. In spite of this skeptical example, the name has been hugely popular since the 12th-century martyrdom of Thomas à Becket. The recent vogue for unusual names has somewhat eclipsed this old standard but it is still one of the basic names for boys born in the United States.

Thom, Thompson, Thomson, Tom, Tomas, Tomaso, Tomasso, Tomasz, Tomkin, Tomlin, Tommaso, Tommy

Thor *ONorse.* "Thunder." The Norse god of thunder, Thor, holds an important place in the Norse pantheon, but in the Anglo-Saxon world the name appears more often in derivative forms, as in **Terrell**.

Thorin, Thorvald, Tor

Tibor *Slavic.* "Sacred place."

Timothy *Gk.* "Honoring God." New Testament name, correspondent with Saint Paul. Scanty use until the 18th century, then increased gradually to the middle of the 20th. After a baby boom peak, it has faded to steady but unspectacular use.

> Tim, Timmy, Timo, Timofeo, Timofey, Timon, Timoteo

Titus *Lat.* Unknown meaning. New Testament character. Use is mostly 18th and 19th centuries. In spite of its sound, it has nothing to do with titans or giants.

> Tito, Titos

Tobias *Heb.* "The Lord is good." Old Testament name that faded after the Puritans used it and was revived in the 19th century. The diminutive, **Toby,** is slightly more common now, though still very unusual.

> Tobey, Tobiah, Tobie, Tobit, Toby

Todd *ME.* "Fox." Used mostly in the 20th century, fashionable for a spell in the 1970s. Still quite steadily used.

> Tod

Tony Diminutive of **Anthony** (*Lat.* "Beyond price"). Used independently only since the middle of the 20th century.

> Toney, Tonie

Travis *OF.* Occupational name: "toll taker." Most common in the United States.

> Traver, Travers, Traviss, Travys

Trent *Lat.* Place name: "gushing waters." Name of an important river in England.

Trenten, Trentin, Trenton

Trevor *Welsh.* "Large homestead." Use expanded outside of Wales in the mid-Victorian era, but the name was most popular in the middle of the 20th century.

Trefor, Trevar, Trever

Trey *ME.* "Three." Related to the French *trois* for "three."

Trai, Traye, Tre

Tristan *Welsh.* The name's Welsh meaning is unclear, but since *triste* is French for "sad," that explanation is often given. In the medieval legends, Tristan is the knight who is in love with Isolde, wife of his uncle. The tale has been told in many forms, including an epic poem by Tennyson and an opera by Wagner. Use peaked in 1996.

Tris, Tristam, Tristram

Troy *Ir. Gael.* "Foot soldier." The name of the famous Greek city where the Trojan wars were fought. Also, a fairly common place name in the United States (as in Troy, NY).

Troi, Troye

Tucker *OE.* Occupational name: "fabric pleater." Another occupational name relating to one of medieval Britain's principal industries, the woolen trade.

Tuck, Tuckerman

Turner *ME.* Occupational name: "wood worker." *Turning* referred to use of a lathe, which provided the decorative elements on much furniture in the 16th and 17th centuries.

Tyler *OE.* Occupational name: "maker of tiles." The name of one of the less memorable presidents in the United States (John Tyler, 1841–1845). Still, the name rocketed up popularity charts in the 1990s, with no clear prompting from popular culture. After a spell in the top 10, it is beginning to drift out of fashion.

> Ty, Tylar

Tyrone *Ir. Gael.* "Land of Owen." Given prominence almost entirely by the actors Tyrone Power Sr. and Jr. around the middle of the 20th century.

> Tyron

Ulric *OG.* "Power of the wolf '' or "power of the home." Used in Britain before the Norman invasion but barely known in the last nine hundred or so years.

> Rick, Udo, Ullric, Ulrich

Ulysses *Lat.* Variation of **Odysseus,** which may mean "wrathful." American use was spurred by the presidency of Civil War hero Ulysses S. Grant. Now rare.

> Ulises, Ulisse

Umberto *It.* Variation of **Humbert** (*OG.* "Renowned hun"). A
royal name in Italy, though very scarce in English-speaking
countries.

Urban *Lat.* "From the city." We have a modern word, *urbane,*
from the same root. Apparently, in ancient times city dwellers had better manners than their rural contemporaries.
Though the name was used by eight popes, it is scarce
today in English-speaking countries.

> Urbain, Urbano, Urbanus

Uriah *Heb.* "The Lord is my light." Prominent Old Testament
name at its most popular in the 19th century, though literary parents will be reminded of the smarmy, hand-wringing
Uriah Heep in Dickens's *David Copperfield.*

> Uri, Urias, Uriyah

Uriel *Heb.* "Flame of God." The Muslim version of the name is
Israfil; he is the Muslim angel of music and appears in the
Koran along with Gabriel and Michael. In Christian terms,
he is one of seven named archangels.

Vail *OE.* Place name: "valley." Famous now as a ski resort in
Colorado. Generally a transferred last name.

> Vaile, Vaill, Vale

291 VICTOR

Valentine *Lat.* "Strong." This name and **Valerian** come from
the same root. Valentine is used for both boys and girls,
although the early Christian martyr for whom the holiday is
named was male.

> Val, Valentijn, Valentin, Valentino

Valerian *Lat.* "Strong, healthy." Far less common than the
feminine version, **Valerie**.

> Valerien, Valerio, Valerius, Valery

Van *Dutch.* "Of." A particle of many Dutch names. Also possibly a nickname for **Evan**. Originally may have been used
as a nickname for children with transferred Dutch last
names, but it became generally popular in the middle of
the 20th century.

> Vann, Von, Vonn

Vance *OE.* Place name: "marshland."

Vanya *Rus.* Diminutive of **John** (*Heb.* "The Lord is gracious")
via **Ivan**. Rare outside of Russia.

Vasilis *Gk.* "Royal, kingly." More familiar in its anglicized form,
Basil.

> Vasily, Vassily, Vasya, Wassily

Vernon *OF.* Place name: "alder grove." A Norman name that
took root as an English last name and, by the 19th century, a first name.

> Vern, Verney

Victor *Lat.* "Conqueror." Extremely common in Christian

Rome, as was its female form, **Victoria.** Revived during
the reign of Queen Victoria and now quite steadily used.

Vic, Victorin, Viktor, Vittorio

Vincent *Lat.* "Conquering." From the same root as **Victor** but
used much more steadily since early Christian days. It has
not suffered neglect, but neither has it ever been truly
popular. Saint Vincent de Paul, a 17th-century priest,
founded an order of missionary brothers, and the Saint
Vincent de Paul Society, an international charitable organization, was founded in his honor in the 19th century.

Vicente, Vince, Vincents, Vincenzo, Vinnie

Virgil *Lat.* Clan name: possibly meaning "staff bearer." (The
staff would have been part of official insignia in ancient
Rome.) The name is usually homage to the Roman author
of the *Aeneid.*

Verge, Vergil, Virgilio

Vito *Lat.* "Alive." Generally used by Italian families. St. Vitus
was an early martyr whose legend held that he could cure
epilepsy and another disorder known as "St. Vitus' dance."

Vitale, Vitaly, Vitas

Vladimir *Slavic.* "Renowned prince."

Vladamir, Vladimeer, Wladimir, Wladymyr

Wade *OE.* Place name: "river ford." Transferred last name with a certain popularity in old Southern families, after Confederate General Wade Hampton.
>   Waddell, Wadell, Wayde

Walden *OE.* Place name: "wooded valley." Could also be another variant of one of the Old German names that include the "Wald-" ("power") element, such as **Walter.** Many literature-loving parents may think of Thoreau's book and the pond *Walden.*
>   Waldenn, Waldi, Waldon

Waldo Diminutive of Waldemar (*OG.* "Renowned ruler"). The "-o" ending is a particularly Germanic diminutive. Possibly also a German place name: "forest meadow."

Walker *OE.* Occupational name: "Cloth-walker." The era that saw the rise of last names was also the great English era of the wool trade, giving us such cloth manufacturing names as **Dyer, Fuller,** and **Weaver.** In that medieval era, workers trod on the wool to cleanse it of impurities.

Wallace *OE.* "Welshman." Originally a Scottish name used to identify foreigners from the South. Like many last names, it was most popular as a first name in the 19th century.
>   Wallach, Wallis, Wally, Walsh, Welch, Welsh

Walter *OG.* "People of power" or "army of power." Norman name that took root strongly in Britain and has been used quite steadily for the last nine hundred years (with the occasional century of neglect). Not particularly fashionable now.

    Gaultier, Gualtiero, Valter, Walt, Walther, Watkins

Ward *OE.* Occupational name: "watchman." Like many of these occupational or place names turned last names, Ward was revived as a first name in the 19th century. It is still somewhat more common as a first name than most other occupational names (**Baker, Smith, Turner,** etc.).

    Warde, Warden

Warner *OG.* "Fighting defender."

    Werner, Wernher

Warren *OE.* "Watchman"; *ME.* "Park warden." A warren was originally an area devoted to breeding game, especially rabbits. By extension, the word is now used to describe human dwellings that resemble the haphazard and over-crowded rabbits' tunnels. As a name, Warren was used in the late 19th century and given a boost by the career of President Warren G. Harding.

    Ware, Waring, Warrin, Warriner

Watson *OE.* "Son of Walter." Last name used as a first name primarily in the 19th century.

Wayne *OE.* Occupational name: "wagon builder or driver." Its period of greatest popularity coincided with the popularity of the actor Marion Morrison, better known as John Wayne.

> **Wain, Wayn**

Wendell *OG.* "Wanderer." Quite rare.

> **Wendall, Wendel**

Wesley *OE.* Place name: "western meadow." Used in honor of John and Charles Wesley, who founded the Methodist Church in the 18th century.

> **Wesly, Westleigh, Westley**

Whitney *OE.* Place name: "white island." Last name that was annexed as a girl's name in the 1980s. It became much more popular for girls than it ever was for boys.

Whittaker *OE.* Place name: "white field." The last part of the name may refer to an acre of land.

> **Whitacker, Whitaker**

Wilbur *OG.* Last name of obscure meaning. E. B. White fans will associate it with the protagonist of *Charlotte's Web*, Wilbur the Pig.

> **Wilber, Willbur**

Wiley *OE.* Place name: "water meadow." Indicates a meadow that would be flooded from time to time.

> **Willey, Wylie**

Wilford *OE.* Place name: "willow ford."

Wilfred *OE.* "Purposeful peace." A name whose two elements are both nouns (in this case, "will" and "peace"), to the confusion of the translator. Neglected after the Norman

invasion but revived in the 19th century to some popularity,
which never spread as far as the United States.

Wilfredo, Wilfrid, Wilfryd, Will, Willfred

Willard *OG.* "Bold will." Most common in the United States,
though far from a household word.

Willerd

William *OG.* "Will-helmet." Another two-noun name, more
often translated as "resolute protection" or the like. Given a
great boost in Norman England by William the Conqueror
and succeeding English kings. Between the 17th and
20th centuries, one of the top handful of boys' names. Its
popularity faded somewhat in the middle of the 20th century, but by the end, it was one of the top two dozen boys'
names in the United States. Currently in the top 10.

**Bill, Billy, Guglielmo, Guillaume, Guillermo,
Liam, Wilhelm, Will, Willem, Willi, Williamson,
Willis, Willy**

Wilson *OE.* "Son of Will." Last name turned first name, possibly in compliment to President Woodrow Wilson.

Willson

Winston *OE.* Place name: "friend's town" or "wine's town."
For modern parents, recalls both English statesman
Winston Churchill and a popular brand of cigarettes.

Winsten, Winstonn, Wynstan, Wynston

Winthrop *OE.* Place name: "friend's village." In the

United States, it hearkens back to the Puritan governor of Massachusetts, John Winthrop, and his numerous Bostonian descendants.

Wolcott *OE.* Place name: "wolf's cottage." Oliver Wolcott of Connecticut signed the Declaration of Independence.

Wolfgang *OG.* "Wolf gait." A very Germanic name that would not be considered by English-speaking parents without the fame of composer Wolfgang Amadeus Mozart.

Woodrow *OE.* "Row by the woods." *Row* could refer to a row of houses or trees or bushes (as in a hedgerow). The name has been given prominence beyond the usual place name by admirers of President Woodrow Wilson.

    Woody

Woody Diminutive of **Woodrow,** and so on. A particularly American name adopted by actor Allen Konigsberg, now better known as Woody Allen.

Wright *OE.* Occupational name: "carpenter." Again, mostly 19th-century use. The astounding feats of aviators Orville and Wilbur Wright apparently did not inspire parents to use their name in homage.

Wyatt *OF.* "Small fighter." Last name occasionally used as a first name but increasingly fashionable in recent years.

    Wiatt, Wye, Wyeth

Wylie *OE.* "Clever, charming, full of wiles."

    Wiley, Wye

Xan Diminutive of **Alexander** (*Gk.* "Defender of mankind").
Xander, Zan, Zander
Xavier *Basque.* "New house." Most often found as a middle name following **Francis,** in honor of St. Francis Xavier, a 16th-century Jesuit missionary who took Christianity to the East Indies and Japan.
Javier, Saviero, Zavier

Yaakov *Heb.* Variation of **Jacob** ("He who supplants").
Yachov, Yakov
Yasir *Arab.* "Well to do."
Yaseer
Yitzhak *Heb.* Variation of **Isaac** ("laughter").
Itzak, Izaak
Yuri *Rus.* Variation of **George** (*Lat.* "Farmer").
Yves *Fr.* Variation of **Ivo** (*OG.* "Yew wood").

Zachariah *Heb.* "The Lord has remembered." Biblical name occurring in both Old and New Testaments. As might be expected, it was revived by the Puritans and found fairly constantly through the 19th century. **Zachary** is the most popular form and reached the top 20 names in the United States in the mid-1990s.

> Zacarias, Zach, Zacharie, Zachary, Zachery, Zack, Zak, Zakarias

Zalman *Heb.* "Peaceable." Another version of **Solomon.**

Zane Derivation and meaning unclear. May be a variation of **John** (*Heb.* "The Lord is gracious") or a version of a Scandinavian last name. Made famous by author Zane Grey, who wrote many novels about the Wild West, among them *Riders of the Purple Sage.*

> Zain, Zayne

Zeke *Heb.* "Strength of God." Diminutive of **Ezekiel.** Ezekiel was an important Old Testament prophet.

EVEN A GENIUS NEEDS A GEM

DARE TO REPAIR PLUMBING
Julie Sussman and
Stephanie Glakas-Tenet
ISBN 0-06-083458-7

MENTAL_FLOSS PRESENTS INSTANT KNOWLEDGE
ISBN 0-06-083461-7

THE 3-HOUR DIET™ ON THE GO
Jorge Cruise
ISBN 0-06-079319-8

EMILY POST'S FAVORITE PARTY & DINING TIPS
Peggy Post
ISBN 0-06-083459-5

PHIL HELLMUTH'S TEXAS HOLD'EM
Phil Hellmuth
ISBN 0-06-083460-9

SAS SURVIVAL HANDBOOK
John 'Lofty' Wiseman
ISBN 0-06-084982-7

QUOTATIONS
ISBN 0-06-081871-9

FENG SHUI
(ON SALE 6/13/06)
Richard Craze
ISBN 0-06-089689-2

TAROT
(ON SALE 6/13/06)
Rowenna Stuart
ISBN 0-06-089688-4

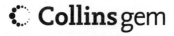
Collins gem